Edited by
ANDREW SIMS

Speech and Language Disorders in Psychiatry

Proceedings of the Fifth Leeds Psychopathology Symposium

GASKELL

©The Royal College of Psychiatrists 1995

Gaskell is an imprint of the Royal College of Psychiatrists,
17 Belgrave Square, London SW1

All rights reserved. No part of this book may be reprinted
or reproduced or utilised in any form or by any electronic,
mechanical, or other means, now known or hereafter invented,
including photocopying and recording, or in any information
storage or retrieval system, without permission in writing
from the publishers.

British Library Cataloguing-in-Publication Data
A catalogue record for this book is available from the British Library

ISBN 0-902241-79-6

Distributed in North America
by American Psychiatric Press, Inc.

ISBN 0-88048-640-6

The views presented in this book do not necessarily
reflect those of the Royal College of Psychiatrists,
and the publishers are not responsible for any error
of omission or fact.

The Royal College of Psychiatrists is a registered charity (no. 228636).

Cover design by Louise Williams/Science Photo Library
Phototypeset by Dobbie Typesetting Ltd, Tavistock, Devon
Printed by Bell & Bain Ltd, Thornliebank, Glasgow

Contents

List of contributors vii

Part I. The background

1 Introduction. The descriptive psychopathology of speech and language *Andrew Sims* 3
2 Disorders of thought and language in psychiatry: a conceptual history *German Berrios* 15
3 Analysis of language: terminology and techniques *David Newby* 31

Part II. Schizophrenic disturbance of speech and language

4 On analysing schizophrenic speech: what model should we use? *Elaine Chaika* 47
5 Language impairments and executive dysfunction in schizophrenia *Rodney Morice* 57
6 Thought, speech and language disorder and semantic memory in schizophrenia *Ann Mortimer, Bryan Corridan, Shauna Rudge, King Kho, Frank Kelly, Michael Bristow and John Hodges* 70
7 Schizophasia: the glossomanic and the glossolalic subtypes *André Roch Lecours* 81
8 Syntactic processing and communication disorder in first-onset schizophrenia *Philip Thomas and Ivan Leudar* 96
9 The psychology of schizophrenic thought; the neuropsychology of schizophrenic speech *Peter McKenna* 113
10 Semantic processing and categorisation in schizophrenia *Eric Chen, Peter McKenna and Arnold Wilkins* 126
11 German concepts of schizophrenic language disorder and reality assessment *Christoph Mundt* 138
12 Thought insertion, insight and Descartes' *cogito*: linguistic analysis and the descriptive psychopathology of schizophrenic thought disorder *K. W. M. Fulford* 147

Part III. Other psychiatric disorders

13 Some aspects of language disorder in dementia *Edgar Miller* 163
14 The semantics of autism *Peter Hobson* 174
15 Growth points in the neurology of speech and language
    E. M. R. Critchley 185

Index 195

Contributors

German Berrios, Consultant and University Lecturer in Psychiatry, Department of Psychiatry, University of Cambridge, Addenbrooke's Hospital, Hills Road, Cambridge CB2 2QQ
Michael Bristow, Senior Registrar, Charing Cross and Westminster Medical School, London
Elaine Chaika, Program in Linguistics, Providence College, Providence, RI 02918, USA
Eric Chen, Department of Psychiatry, Addenbrooke's Hospital, Hills Road, Cambridge
Brian Corridan, Registrar, Charing Cross and Westminster Medical School, London
E. M. R. Critchley, Consultant Neurologist, Honorary Professor of Neurology, University of Central Lancashire, Royal Preston Hospital, Preston, Lancashire PR2 4HT
K. W. M. Fulford, Honorary Consultant Psychiatrist, Research Fellow, Green College Oxford; University Department of Psychiatry, Warneford Hospital, Oxford OX3 7JX
Peter Hobson, Professor, Developmental Psychopathology Research Unit, Tavistock Clinic, 120 Belsize Lane, London NW3 5BA, and Department of Psychiatry, University College, London
John Hodges, Lecturer in Psychiatry, University of Cambridge, Cambridge
Frank Kelly, Registrar, Charing Cross and Westminster Medical School, London
King Kho, Registrar, Charing Cross and Westminster Medical School, London
André Roch Lecours, Centre de recherche du Centre hospitalier Côte-des-Neiges 4565, chemin Queen Mary, Montréal, Canada H3W 1W5
Ivan Leudar, Department of Psychology, University of Manchester, Coupland Street, off Oxford Road, Manchester M13

Peter McKenna, Consultant Psychiatrist, Fulbourn Hospital, Cambridge CB1 5EF

Edgar Miller, Professor of Clinical Psychology, Department of Psychology, University of Leicester, Leicester LE1 7RH

Rodney Morice, Director of Mental Health Services, Department of Health, South-West Health Districts of New South Wales, 481 George Street, Albury, New South Wales 2640, Australia

Ann Mortimer, Senior Lecturer in Psychiatry, Charing Cross and Westminster Medical School, London, c/o West London Healthcare NHS Trust, Uxbridge Road, Southall, Middlesex UB1 3EU

Christoph Mundt, Director, Psychiatrische Klinik, Ruprecht-Karls-Universität Heidelberg, Voßstraße 4, 69115 Heidelberg, Germany

David Newby, Consultant Psychiatrist, High Royds Hospital, Menston, Ilkley, Yorkshire, and Senior Clinical Lecturer, University of Leeds

Shauna Rudge, Registrar, Charing Cross and Westminster Medical School, London

Andrew Sims, Professor of Psychiatry, Division of Psychiatry and Behavioural Sciences, St James's University Hospital, Leeds LS9 7TF

Philip Thomas, Consultant Psychiatrist and Honorary Clinical Tutor, Community Mental Health Team, Brony Garth Hospital, Penrhyndeudraeth, Gwynedd LL48 6HD

Arnold Wilkins, Senior Research Scientist, MRC Applied Psychology Unit, Cambridge

Part I. The background

1 Introduction. The descriptive psychopathology of speech and language

ANDREW SIMS

"Words are truly people, magic people, having birth, growth and destiny."
John Steinbeck

Communication, and its study, is an essential part of psychiatry. It is through sounds, mostly words, that patients are able to tell us about their symptoms and reveal the signs of illness. The absence of speech is a symptom in itself. The doctor, also, uses words for communication, both in making inquiry in a psychiatric history, and in establishing a therapeutic relationship. Speech is a window for the mind.

The speech of the patient informs both about symptoms – the nature of the complaint and the subjective experience of distress – and about signs – the evidence to an outside observer that there is psychiatric disorder, whether or not the patient is aware of it as a complaint.

There are considerable differences in the abnormalities of speech in the major psychiatric diagnostic groups. Organic psychosyndromes, for example, may be manifested particularly in abnormality of articulation, in some type of dysphasia, or in an altered state of consciousness resulting in diminished speech. A large part of this book is devoted to abnormalities of speech and language in schizophrenia; although these are very varied, there are common patterns. Peculiarities in the nature of speech behaviour are characteristic of both mania and depression, among affective disorders; retardation and poverty of association are characteristic of depression, and multiple associations are related to weakening of the determining tendency (the consistent direction of thinking towards its goal), and hence pressure of speech and flight of ideas are characteristic of mania. In neurotic disorders, the abnormality is more with the content of speech, with the disturbance in self-image and in the experience of relationships.

The study of speech and language disorder gives information not only about this particular psychopathological function but also about other areas of disturbance. For this reason, the Fifth Leeds Psychopathology Symposium was devoted to the study of speech and language disorders in psychiatry. Previous symposia had looked at other psychopathological functions, including the psychopathology of depression, the psychopathology of body image (Rix & Snaith, 1988), disorders of perception (Sims, 1991*a*), and delusions and awareness of reality (Sims, 1991*b*). Evaluating symptoms according to their psychopathological function has resulted in well-known phenomena of mental illness being viewed from a different perspective; research and therapeutic ideas are thereby stimulated in a different manner compared with starting from the traditional standpoint of individual psychiatric disorders. It is the intention, when possible, to link the phenomena of descriptive psychopathology to known abnormalities in neurobiology and experimental psychology; combining these three different approaches holds advantages for our psychiatric understanding. Knowledge acquired from discussing these different psychopathological functions consecutively – body image, perception, delusions, speech – is cumulative; how this can be developed into a composite theory will be described later in this chapter for the psychopathology of schizophrenia.

Speech and language in psychiatry: the background

It is appropriately within the tradition of descriptive psychopathology that our scrutiny of speech and language disorder in psychiatry should begin with German Berrios' conceptual analysis on the history of ideas concerning thought and language in psychiatry (Chapter 2). This is the logical starting place, or, as he quotes Macevoy: "it may be said that we know nothing absolutely concerning any question if we ignore its beginning". During the 19th century, as both psychiatry as a separate discipline and the study of thinking and speaking were developing, two models for thinking were dominant. These were associationism, based on Locke's theory of simple and complex ideas, considering that the process of thinking was a linking of separate ideas, and faculty psychology, in which the mind was conceived as a cluster of independent faculties, and differing faculties, such as the intellect, could even have specific locations in the brain.

Berrios develops the history of the origins of psychiatric views on thought and language through earlier authors into the 19th century; he discusses the work of Hughlings Jackson (with his significant Yorkshire associations); and especially concentrates on the important but little-known work of Séglas, who divided disorders of speech and language into pathology of thought (*dyslogie*), of language (*dysphasie*), and of speech (*dyslalie*). Masselon's views on thought disorder in dementia praecox have also been generally neglected, and their significance for current understanding is shown. Our present lack of clarity and conflicting conceptualisations of speech and language disorders only repeat classic arguments that preceded modern psychiatry and psychology.

For achieving an understanding of the thought, speech and language disorders of their patients, psychiatrists have to understand something of the scientific bases and methods of analysis of language itself; mostly, however, they have no academic foundation in the study of language, nor knowledge of psycholinguistics upon which to do this. In Chapter 3, David Newby sets out to make this topic intelligible for psychiatrists who have a background knowledge of psychopathology but not of psycholinguistics. He develops the theme that speech does not necessarily precisely mirror thought, and the relationship between these two are explored. The analysis carried out by linguistics, with definitions and examples of technical terms, is illustrated with relevant case material from psychiatry.

Schizophrenic disturbance of speech and language

Within the study of speech and language disorders in psychiatry, much more attention has been paid to schizophrenia, and to the evidence of thought disorder of schizophrenic subjects, than to any other condition. The reasons for this are that the thinking processes, as evinced by speech of schizophrenic patients, is clearly disordered; it conforms to certain constantly recurring patterns which hold the challenge of accurate description and analysis; and, up to now, it has not been possible to apply a linguistic or neuropsychological model that truly fits all sufferers from the condition. Hence most attention is given in this book to the study of schizophrenia. The authors approach their subject from different disciplines and standpoints, and come to different conclusions. The distillate of collective knowledge, obtained from both experiment and the observation of individuals, helps us to a greater understanding of the subjective experience and thinking process of the schizophrenic patient.

Elaine Chaika develops the argument that language responds to cognitive and pragmatic forces, and that it is here, rather than merely in syntactic generation, that the abnormalities of schizophrenia should be sought; in fact, in the usage of patients and normal people alike, there is *speech*, which is functional, but no purely abstract *language*. There is no disruption in basic language competence in schizophrenia and yet speech is clearly disordered and incoherent. It is proposed that, rather than looking for particular disorder of syntax in schizophrenic speech, recent investigations into slips of the tongue and the architecture of volition may offer better models for exploring schizophrenia. Schizophrenic patients may be demonstrating particularly severe slip-of-the-tongue phenomena, which, however, unlike normal subjects, they do not recognise or identify on replaying tapes of their own speech. The error of schizophrenic speech is in executive control rather than just linguistic dysfunction, according to this theory.

Both Kraepelin and Bleuler pointed out abnormalities in the speech of schizophrenic patients; Kraepelin was more concerned with possible anatomical lesions following the neuroanatomical localisations of Broca and Wernicke, while Bleuler concentrated upon conceptual thought disorder and its manifestation in speech. Rodney Morice links these dichotomous approaches in Chapter 5, in a report of his work involving a computer-assisted analysis of manually parsed samples of free speech from schizophrenic subjects; syntax tree diagrams were produced for each analysable sentence. The interpretation of results from this method would suggest that language impairment in schizophrenia could result from executive dysfunction, especially impairment of working memory, rather than specific language dysfunction similar to that resulting from damage in either Broca's or Wernicke's areas. This impairment in schizophrenia could be part of a more general 'dysexecutive syndrome' mediated in the prefrontal cortex.

Ann Mortimer points out that there may also be mechanical reasons for the difficulty in understanding the speech of schizophrenic patients: orofacial dyskinesia, oversedation, slurring, missing or badly fitting teeth causing dysarthria, or aprosodic speech with unusual tone or rhythm. There are some similarities between receptive aphasia and schizophrenic speech, but also considerable differences, of which the absence of insight concerning a disability in schizophrenia is prominent. Two studies with schizophrenic patients are reported. In the first, semantic memory was assessed with the 'silly sentences test', in which many schizophrenic patients said that the silly sentences were true. In the second, using Hodges' semantic battery, the majority of patients appeared to show problems with semantic access and manipulation, while some may also have had semantic store disorder, with poverty of thought.

In Chapter 7, André Roch Lecours discusses the speech of schizophrenic patients showing glossomanic and/or glossolalic abnormalities. He shows how glossomanic speech differs essentially from the 'jargon aphasia' of Wernicke's syndrome, for example, by breaking standard phonological conventions. Glossolalic speech uses a tiny lexicon of word-like units – "far smaller than that of a standard dolphin". Glossomania has more in common with certain forms of literary creation than with fluent aphasia; it is probably not only associated with schizophrenia. The glossolalia of schizophrenia is episodic (conventional speech also occurs), and is produced as a monologue which mimics stereotyped speech. Lecours demonstrates the benefits of detailed consideration of the surprising and unexpected words and phrases actually used by schizophrenic patients.

There are some advantages in using written language to study the abnormalities of psychosis; it is free of the immediate social context and may therefore be more sensitive to the direct effects of language processing and changes in cognition. Philip Thomas and Ivan Leudar (Chapter 8) studied such material using the Hunt test, in which subjects are asked to rewrite, more concisely, 32 propositions in the form of simple sentences, comparing thought-disordered subjects with those without thought disorder among first-onset schizophrenic patients. Their findings suggest that communication disorder in acute schizophrenia is associated with a specific disorder of language processing, and is *not* dependent upon other aspects of cognition; more syntactical errors occur with more complex tasks.

Formal thought disorder is one of the few signs in schizophrenia, according to Peter McKenna (Chapter 9). However, among psychological investigations of formal thought disorder, only overinclusive thinking has proved to be a fairly robust finding. Schizophrenic speech contains less redundancy than normal speech, is less predictable, and contains less information. Studies of the neuropsychology of language, although showing deficits in schizophrenic patients, have not indicated any specific abnormality beyond the overall level of intellectual impairment. In chronic schizophrenia, intellectual impairment has become more marked and sometimes the speech disorder is more obviously dysphasic.

Categorisation tasks have proved a satisfactory way of assessing semantic memory. Schizophrenic patients were slow at completing such tasks and showed a consistent pattern of response; they were overinclusive in semantic categories. This may be due to excessive 'priming' in relation to semantic tasks by schizophrenic patients which alters the nature of decision made. According to Eric Chen *et al* (Chapter 10), the semantic categories in schizophrenia are intact internally, but the category boundaries are expanded; this has implications for the interaction between working memory and semantic memory.

Thought and language disorder has been investigated extensively in German psychiatry, following the association studies of Kraepelin, Aschaffenburg and Bleuler at the end of the 19th century and early in the 20th. In Chapter 11, Christoph Mundt considers that the interest then subsided, to be rediscovered by the anthropological phenomenology of the 1960s and the concurrent possibility of objectifying and quantifying abnormal phenomena. More recently, Blankenburg has localised, conceptually, the disturbance of thought and speech in schizophrenia in the moving back and forth between preverbal and verbal thinking. In being pre-predicative, delusions are judgements which are not subject to interpersonal agreement. Normal communication implies intact ego boundaries; this is disturbed in schizophrenia. Concretism and reification of words may be vested in some sort of magical power in schizophasia. German psychopathological studies of the last 40 years do not investigate thought and language as isolated phenomena, but as a means to exploring more general disturbance in self and relationship.

In Chapter 12, K. W. M. Fulford links and contrasts Descartes' notion of *"cogito ergo sum"* – "I think therefore I am" – with the fundamental schizophrenic symptom of thought insertion – thinking *other people's* thoughts. He considers that thought insertion should be of interest to philosophers and the *cogito* to psychopathologists. The principle of adhesiveness is important – not only for thoughts but for any conscious experience – and it is this that is lost in thought insertion. The oddness and uniqueness of the symptom of thought insertion, and how this relates to the much maligned but still useful psychotic/non-psychotic dichotomy, are emphasised. The philosophical understanding of insight is relevant for this discussion, and this can be used to examine psychiatric concepts. Psychopathology can become a resource for philosophy on the principle that discoveries tend to follow explanations for things going wrong, rather than where mechanisms are functioning smoothly; the study of thought insertion is a good example of this. With thought insertion, 'I think' becomes detached from the ownership of that thought, and yet the separation of 'I' and 'think' in thought insertion shows that 'I think' does imply 'I am'.

All these authors are agreed that common-sense observation and clinical experience put the group of patients diagnosed as suffering from schizophrenia into a category of their own, separate and distinguishable in general terms from normal health, from other broad psychiatric diagnostic groupings, and from organic disorders of the brain manifesting in the dysphasic disorders; there are quantitative diagnostic criteria for identifying sufferers from schizophrenia. Authors are also agreed that the speech of many schizophrenic patients is grossly disordered, that there are abnormalities of language, and that these together point to disturbance in the thinking process. The relationship between thought and speech disorder, which of these two is causative or whether both are secondary to another factor, is complex and has given rise to much argument and speculation.

Many of the tests used for investigating speech and language demonstrate abnormality in schizophrenia. To what extent are schizophrenic patients abnormal? Is this abnormality specific for schizophrenia, or is it found in other conditions? What does it tell us about the underlying psychopathology of schizophrenia? We are reminded that there may be non-specific abnormalities of articulation in schizophrenia and also eccentricities of pitch and rhythm. Abnormalities have been described in both syntax and semantics among schizophrenic patients.

Other psychiatric disorders

There are many potential pitfalls in the study of language impairment in Alzheimer-type dementia. Errors in naming, which are especially prominent, may be partially but not wholly caused by faulty perception; there is also a strong semantic component. Conversational speech also, according to Edgar Miller (Chapter 13), is impoverished, less elaborate and more fragmented. Problems with comprehension occur; lexical difficulties appear to be the major problem for written material, and there are problems in understanding familiar idiomatic phrases. Most language-related activities show some impairment and there is a tendency to perseverate verbal responses. However, the language disorder of Alzheimer's disease, unlike cerebrovascular dementia, does not seem to be qualitatively the same as that found in any of the aphasic syndromes with focal lesions. Syntax and phonological aspects of language are relatively well preserved in Alzheimer's disease.

Autism is a syndrome with early onset comprising disorder of social interaction and communication, social imagination and understanding, and associated with repetitive patterns of behaviour and unusual responses to stimuli. In Chapter 14, Peter Hobson relates this to the normal development of interpersonal understanding that occurs before the development of language in the second year of life. Part of the 'essence' of autism is the subjective experience of the observer in being treated like a piece of furniture; there is a failure, in the condition, in interpersonal, especially affective, engagement, and in the capacity for intersubjective coordination. When autistic subjects were compared with mentally retarded and normal subjects, they were found to have a specific disability in naming emotions, and were also specifically poorer at identifying emotion-related items from pictures. There is a defect in autism in the use of personal pronouns, and this often results in the inappropriate use of proper names. Language affords valuable insights into the nature of the impoverished interpersonal world of the autistic patient, and autism may well illuminate some of the origins and nature of language itself.

For the scientific study of speech and language disorder in neurology, E. M. R. Critchley (Chapter 15) considers it essential to differentiate receptive disorders, especially deafness, from disorders of comprehension. Listening, however, also involves looking – for example, evaluating the facial expression of the speaker. Central disorders of language may be misdiagnosed as simple deafness. Some speech-related activities are associated with the non-dominant hemisphere, such as prosody, reading rather than speech, and some supralinguistic functions such as word-finding. Otherwise, lateralisation of speech shows most functions to be based in the dominant hemisphere. Aphasias should not be seen as static but dynamic conditions which change over time, with localisation affecting their nature; it is also apparent that lesions in the same area may result in different abnormalities. The frontal lobes exert an influence on speech by regulating, controlling, programming and executing activity and sequences of actions.

Speech and language disorder in schizophrenia and the permeability of self

Much of this book is taken up with exploring the separate strands of the many investigations which have been carried out into the disordered speech and language of patients suffering from schizophrenia. The abnormalities of speech in dementia and in neurological conditions manifesting as dysphasia can be contrasted with schizophrenia and, without any very elaborate investigation, large differences become apparent. The specific language disorder of autism differs significantly from schizophrenia in that the abnormality of autism ultimately lies in interpersonal relationship, while much of the evidence for schizophrenia would point to an abnormality of self-image.

Much of the work on perceptual abnormalities in schizophrenia, especially auditory hallucinations, would suggest that the disturbed and altered new *meaning* is of much more significance to the patient than any possible change in the nature of perception itself; a cognitive account of hallucination would suggest that an internal event is inferred to be an outside event (Bentall, 1990). Similarly, delusions in schizophrenia always have specific meaning for the patient. This was well exemplified by Roberts (1991), who described how the gross and bizarre delusions of patients with chronic schizophrenia gave the patients themselves a new sense of identity, a clearer sense of duty and responsibility, often an experience of freedom and protection from past hurts, and an affective change away from fear, worry, depression and boredom towards feeling lively, enthusiastic, interested and peaceful. Thus, investigations of areas of the psychopathology of schizophrenia other than thought and speech would suggest major abnormalities in the way subjects view themselves, and their interpretation of events going on outside, in relation to what is happening inside themselves.

Jaspers (1963) categorised the modes in which the self becomes aware of itself in terms of four formal characteristics: the feeling of activity, an awareness of unity, awareness of identity, and awareness of the self as distinct from an outer world and all that is not the self. All four of these functions may be disturbed in the course of a schizophrenic illness but the last of these – which has also been described as permeability of the barrier between the individual and the environment, or loss of ego boundaries (Schneider, 1957) – appears to show some degree of specificity. There is disorder of the boundaries of self, a sense of invasion of self, and merging between self and not self – according to Jaspers (1963), loss of ''the clear sense of the self confronting an outside world . . . cancellation of the distinction we normally draw between the self and the outside world''.

The symptoms of first rank of schizophrenia ascribed to Kurt Schneider (1939) are as follows:

(a) audible thoughts
(b) voices heard arguing
(c) voices heard commenting on one's actions
(d) the experience of influences playing on the body (somatic passivity experiences)

(e) thought withdrawal and other interference with thought
(f) diffusion of thought
(g) delusional perception
(h) all feelings and impulses (drives) are experienced by the patient as the work or influence of others.

A detailed examination of the descriptive psychopathology of these symptoms as they present in schizophrenic patients shows that a disorder of permeability of self occurs in all of them; that is, the presence of first-rank symptoms may be seen as a reasonably specific indicator of disturbance in the boundaries of self (Sims, 1993).

The symptom of thought insertion, as occurs in schizophrenia, and discussed by Fulford, is a symptom of first rank, and was classified by Schneider within "thought withdrawal and other interference with thought". Phenomenologically, in terms of the subjective description of self-experience of the sufferer, it is not essentially different from the other situations where people describe their thoughts as being interfered with: "My thoughts, which are inside my head, my brain, my mind and which I thought were entirely under my own control, are actually being added to by insertion, taken out of me, influenced by others, broadcast to others by an outside source." That is, what I had assumed to be the very most 'inside me' and 'essentially me' and under my own control, the possession of my own thoughts and what I choose to think, I find has actually become 'outside'. It is, therefore, very easy to see how thought insertion represents permeability of boundaries of the self – thinking, which was thought to be taking place within the frontiers of the self, has been invaded from outside, so that self is thinking other people's thoughts.

An example of thought insertion occurring with other schizophrenic symptoms and demonstrating permeability of self was offered by a girl, aged 20, from an Asian country. Her illness began after her best friend persuaded her to have boyfriends. Her friend told her that she should have a 'special boyfriend' and encouraged her to look around for boys who were still without a girlfriend. She noted that a classmate, SR, had no girlfriend and told this to her best friend, not realising that she was making fun of her. Her friend told others about her interest in SR and they started to tease her and make jokes about it. She felt very embarrassed and began to feel that SR was influencing her. In her room she began to see lights and images and felt that someone was watching her. She believed that when she was watching television, the programmes were related to her and when she attended lectures, they related to her also; for example, when the lecturer talked about communal law, she considered that it was her that the lecturer was referring to. She came to accept that everything was planned for and focused upon her. She felt that it was part of the big plan to get married to SR. "They directed it at me." She started to hear the voice of her friend telling her that SR liked her and once, while having a conversation with her friend, she believed that her friend had put something into her mind to make her like SR. She also began to hear SR's voice and could communicate with him through her mind. She began to dress to please SR. Then she heard voices telling her "to phone SR" and she telephoned him asking him whether it was true that he wanted to marry her. SR said that it was not true and said: "You are acting strangely sitting at the back and never talking and never studying".

It is claimed by Mundt, on the basis of the German tradition of psychopathology, that normal communication implies intact boundaries of the self and that these are disturbed in schizophrenia. This would suggest that not only may perceptual abnormalities – such as auditory hallucinations, and more specifically hearing one's thoughts aloud, hearing voices arguing, and hearing voices commenting on one's actions, and also delusions, such as delusions of control – manifest the disturbance in boundaries of self in schizophrenia, but thought and language disorder may also have this as its underlying abnormality. This could link the discrepant findings of many of the studies of this book, and explain the consistent finding that the semantic abnormality seems to be more important than syntactic disturbance. Chaika, for instance, emphasises the cognitive and pragmatic forces that result in schizophrenic abnormalities as exemplified by investigation into slips of the tongue. Why is it that normal individuals when hearing their speech recorded with slips of the tongue recognise the abnormality, but schizophrenic patients do not? Perhaps they still attach to the seemingly neutral statement or situation the abnormal, self-related meaning, and hence expression, initially injected. In the same way that slips of the tongue have been investigated by psychoanalysts for the areas of conflict and self-involvement of neurotic subjects, so also they may indicate self-reference in schizophrenia.

Perhaps executive dysfunction, with its implications for the impairment of working memory (Chapter 5), could also demonstrate the difficulties that patients have in keeping their own self-referent notions out of responses to supposedly objective, neutral questions. The more complex the task, the more likely is the self-concept to become permeable, and therefore errors in test material become increasingly frequent. This is a possible explanation for the abnormalities that Mortimer describes with the 'silly sentences test' with schizophrenic patients. For example, the patient who agreed with the statement "Captains are used for eating soup" offered the explanation, "To feed with – soup. I think they eat soup don't they, they don't get hungry – use him with a spoon". It is possible, although by no means proven, that the variable use of pronouns indicates some injection of self by the patient into the nonsensical and objective statement of the test, and that this has accounted for the error. Again, the absence of insight concerning the abnormality would indicate that the subject 'really meant' the response.

The problem with semantic access and manipulation may be caused by the continuing permeability of self-boundaries. It is useful to look at the unexpected words used by schizophrenic patients and to see if permeability of self could have contributed to their selection.

Why is it that overinclusive thinking, for instance, is not universally apparent in schizophrenic thought and speech, but only on certain occasions? Perhaps it is only on those occasions when the self-concept has intruded. This might explain McKenna's reference to a clarinet by a patient as "wheel support . . . man . . . animal". Perhaps when the object is not recognised, the scope for intrusion and permeability becomes greater. In the terms of the chapter by Chen *et al*, 'priming' may have already occurred in schizophrenic subjects, inasmuch as the semantics of significant ideas may already be 'primed' by notions of self-concept that the patient has brought into the test situation from everyday experiences. Thus, an individual sufferer from schizophrenia may already be predisposed to give an abnormal response to a particular and specific stimulus in a test situation; the category boundaries have been expanded by incorporation of elements of the self into that category which would, logically, be self-neutral.

The hypothesis is that the schizophrenic subject has been unable to keep what should normally be internal and private elements of the self out of dialogue concerning the whole of the rest of life, and so speech and language become contaminated. It is perhaps rather like the chef's tie dipping in the soup; it has not been possible to keep self and its appendages entirely separate from everything else outside, which is not self. It is not impossible that permeability of self, the integrity of self, and its clear distinction from not self, might be a single, yet highly complex, neuropsychological function, perhaps analogous to colour blindness in being a single function represented at different neuroanatomical sites. McKenna (1987) has demonstrated a relationship between brain localisation in schizophrenia and various of the psychopathological symptoms. It could be that disturbance of the boundaries of self could be linked neuropathologically with a limbic lesion in the dominant hemisphere. Such a hypothesis is at present merely conjectural, but a linking theory such as this can explain some of the different findings coming from research into speech and language disorder, and can also relate them to other psychopathological functions, such as disturbance in perception, and delusion.

Conclusions

Speech reveals thought, and disturbed mental functioning is manifested in abnormalities of thinking. Thus the study of speech and language gives valuable insights into the psychopathology of many psychiatric disorders. In order to study speech and language disorder it is important to see how the concepts used have been developed, and also to understand the basic terms and ideas of psycholinguistics.

Much of this book is devoted to the study of schizophrenic speech, language and thought disorder from several different experimental approaches. A unifying hypothesis could be the disturbance in the permeability of self, and loss of ego boundaries, in schizophrenia. This has been shown to be present in schizophrenic auditory hallucinations, delusions, and in all those symptoms regarded by Schneider as being of first rank. The awareness of self, as distinct from an outer world and all that is not the self, could represent a single neuropsychological function which has been damaged in schizophrenic patients.

There are abnormalities of speech and language in Alzheimer's disease, autism and the organic, neurological conditions resulting in dysphasia. Knowledge of linguistics contributes to the understanding of these conditions, and unravelling their distinctive psychopathology gives greater insight into the structure and development of language itself.

References

BENTALL, R. P. (1990) The illusion of reality: a review and integration of psychological research on hallucinations. *Psychological Bulletin*, **107**, 82-95.
JASPERS, K. (1963) *General Psychopathology* (7th edn) (trans. J. Hoenig & M. W. Hamilton). Manchester: Manchester University Press.
MCKENNA, P. J. (1987) Pathology, phenomenology and the dopamine hypothesis of schizophrenia. *British Journal of Psychiatry*, **151**, 288-301.
RIX, K. J. B. & SNAITH, R. P. (1988) The psychopathology of body image. *British Journal of Psychiatry*, **153** (suppl. 2).
ROBERTS, G. (1991) Delusional belief systems and meaning in life: a preferred reality. *British Journal of Psychiatry*, **159** (suppl. 14), 19-28.
SCHNEIDER, K. (1939) Psychischer Befund und Psychiatrische Diagnose. In *Clinical Psychopathology* (M. W. Hamilton, 1959). New York: Grune & Stratton.
—— (1957) Primary and secondary symptoms in schizophrenia (trans. H. Marshall). In *Themes and Variations in European Psychiatry: An Anthology* (eds S. R. Hirsch & M. Shepherd, 1974). Charlottesville: University Press of Virginia.
SIMS, A. C. P. (1991a) An overview of the psychopathology of perception: first rank symptoms as a localising sign in schizophrenia. *Psychopathology*, **24**, 369-374.
—— (1991b) *Delusions and Awareness of Reality: Proceedings of the Fourth Leeds Psychopathology Symposium*. British Journal of Psychiatry, **159** (suppl. 14).
—— (1993) Schizophrenia and permeability of self. *Neurology, Psychiatry and Brain Research*, **1**, 133-135.

2 Disorders of thought and language in psychiatry: a conceptual history

GERMAN BERRIOS

In October 1892, an anonymous British reviewer wrote of Séglas' classic work *Des Troubles du Langage chez les Aliénés* that: "it is remarkable that so few have occupied themselves with this study except in the case of general paralysis" (*Journal of Mental Science*, 1892). He was right. Although the second half of the 19th century teems with work on aphasia and other disorders of language and communcation, little had until then been written on the disorders of language in the mentally ill. This fact is the more curious for the 19th century was, in a general sense, obsessed with the study of language; indeed, it was the period when many grand hypotheses were put forward on its origin and evolution. John Macevoy (1900), a minor Scottish alienist, expressed such sentiment well: "it may be said that we know nothing absolutely concerning any question if we ignore its beginning". He was referring to the historicist approach that was to prove so useful to 19th-century scholars, and which led to important breakthroughs such as evolutionary theory (on historicism, see Iggers, 1973).

In the area of language, the historicist method worked partially. Bopp, Grimm, and particularly Schleicher, conceived of language as a "natural organism with an existence independent from its users" (Leroy, 1969), and this biological metaphor made time and evolution essential to its understanding. Men like Victor Hugo also believed that "the word, remember it, is a living being" (Hugo, 1856), and Cerise proposed the view that language played a crucial role in attaching the "individual organism to collective life, down to the very roots of his material being" (Starobinski, 1974, p. 361).

The unbridled use of the historicist approach caused a glut of hypotheses accounting for the origin of language. This led to a decision by the new Société de Linguistique de Paris (founded in 1866) not to accept papers on the topic (Société de Linguistique de Paris, 1868). By the end of the century, historicist, or *diachronic*, accounts were being complemented (or replaced) by *synchronic*, or static, models of language. Doubtless, the most influential of these was Ferdinand de Saussure's, who began to lecture on it in 1891 in Geneva. Not surprisingly, he had become a member of the Société Linguistique de Paris in 1876 (Koerner, 1982). When writing on the clinical aspects of language during the 19th century, it is tempting to concentrate on the nascent concept of aphasia, and related ideas on brain localisation. But since this area has been chronicled ad nauseam, there is little point in rehearsing its history again except, perhaps, when it is of direct relevance to the history of language disorders *in psychiatry* (for primary sources see Hécaen & Dubois (1969); for classic accounts Moutier (1908) and Marx (1966); and for historiographic pitfalls Bujosa (1980)).

Any account of the history of language disorders in psychiatry must pay attention to three areas:

(a) 19th-century *psychological* views on the relationship between thought and language (particularly those which were influential among alienists)
(b) views on the distinction between neurological and mental disease
(c) theories of language disorder in the *insane*.

For reasons of space, this chapter deals only with (c), by comparing two great and neglected works by Séglas and Masselon. The history of formal thought disorder is also touched upon, as it is clear that during this period the two concepts are inextricably linked. It will be concluded that some of the current tensions and contradictions in the analysis of language disorder in the psychoses (e.g. schizophrenia) can be traced back to the inconclusive debates that took place at the turn of the century. Also for reasons of space, the chapter exclusively focuses on matters clinical, and says nothing on Wundt, Vygotsky, Wittgenstein, Austin, and other men whose contributions to the relationship between thought and language are well known.

Nineteenth-century psychiatric views on thinking and language

Two models of 'thinking' vied for supremacy during the 19th century (Garnier, 1852; Porter, 1868; Taine, 1871; Paulhan, 1889; Dauzat, 1912). One, the legacy of British empiricism, had started with Locke's description of simple and complex ideas: the former directly supported by sensations, the latter resulting from 'reflection'. Thinking linked ideas together by means of laws of association. Associationism, the name under which this theory came to be known (Claparède, 1903; Warren, 1921), inspired theories of thought and its disorders well into the 20th century (e.g. those of Kraepelin and Bleuler – see below).

A second model of thinking emerged from faculty psychology. According to this view, intermittently available since Greek times (Blakey, 1850), the mind was a cluster of independent powers, capacities or faculties, one of which concerned thinking or the processing of information. Partly as a reaction against associationism, versions of faculty psychology were resuscitated by Kant (Hilgard, 1980) and by the Scottish philosophers of common sense (Brooks, 1976). For example, the views of Reid and Stewart were influential among phrenologists (Spoerl, 1936), some of whom went as far as saying that the 'intellectual faculties' were sited in the frontal part of the brain (Spurzheim, 1826; Combe, 1873).

Clinicians aware of these debates, such as Bouillaud (1825), supported the view that human beings possessed a centre for the 'articulation' of language (animals only had the organs of phonation) through which their 'capacity' or faculty to express and understand ideas was exercised. Thus, Bouillaud distinguished 'inner' language from word articulation. The first of these was used by Baillarger (1865) to explain the difference between aphasia without and with preserved capacity to write: in the former, the most likely explanation was 'amnesia'; in the latter, Baillarger suggested, there had been preservation of 'involuntary verbal excitation' with loss of 'voluntary verbal excitation'. If one is to believe Hughlings Jackson (who was given to acknowledge writers he had not followed – such as Spencer – and did not quote those who had really influenced him – like Clifford), the notion of a 'control centre' put forward by Bouillaud and Baillarger was the source of his notion of 'propositional speech', and Baillarger's 'involuntary excitation' of his view on 'automatic speech' (Jackson, 1932, footnote p. 171).

Equally important is the work of Jacques Lordat (1843), who offered one of the earliest 'cascade-type' of accounts of the psychology of language. Focusing on the psychological processes underlying the generation of speech, and based on his own illness (transient aphasia), Lordat conceived of language as a chain of events starting with the identification and description of a concept, and continuing with its parsing out and mapping in memory onto sound and syntactic rules, and concluding in its final execution. Because the model was not dependent upon anatomical knowledge (i.e. it was truly 'conceptual'), it could be used both by alienists to understand thought disorder and by neurologists to explain aphasia.

The relationship between thought and language

Late in the 18th century, Condillac, Rousseau, and Herder worked out a compromise view of the relationship between language and thought:

> "language and thought were interdependent in their development; one could not advance if the other ceased to progress. If, as philosophers believed, the entire process of thought depends upon language, then it followed that to arrive at truths with any precision, language must be extremely accurate." (Juliard,

1970, pp. 45–46) (on this crucial topic also see Cassirer, 1929; Marx, 1966; Raub, 1988)

Belief in the interdependence of thought and language continued well into the 19th century, particularly in the work of Max Müller, who also suggested that language derived "not from shrieks, but from roots, i.e. from general ideas" (Müller, 1882). (This view was to cause a clash between Müller and Darwin; Knoll, 1986.) Müller believed that thought and language were inseparable, and that they could not exist without each other. This belief remained popular until the end of the century (e.g. Moncalm, 1900).

Likewise, during this period it was the rule for alienists to treat disorders of language and thought *together* (even after disorders such as aphasia, aphemia, and alalia had been 'officially' separated). Thus, Falret (1866) reported patients as aphasic who, in fact, were suffering from formal thought disorder and 'nervous' and reversible pathologies of language.

Early descriptions of thought disorder

Around the early 19th century, aphasics, insane patients talking nonsense (Fournier-Pescay & Bégin, 1821) and subjects with disorders of articulation such as stammerers (Rockey, 1980; O'Neill, 1980) were not fully differentiated on conceptual grounds. For example, in his *Commentary on Apoplectic and Paralytic Affections*, Kirkland (1792) reported cases with strokes who "can not get their words out" together with others who had "temporary loss" (p. 158) of the power of speech; and in his major work on the semiology of physical and mental disorders, Landre-Beauvais (1813) dealt with disorders of phonation, speech and language under one heading. Likewise, in their classic entry on *parole*, Fournier-Pescay & Bégin classified the *lesions des organs de la parole* into those resulting from bad habit (*habitudes vicieuses*), congenital disorders (*vices de conformation*), and diseases affecting tissue or its connections (*affections de leurs tissus*) (Fournier-Pescay & Bégin, 1821, p. 329).

This continued until the middle of the century. For example, Snell (1852) drew attention to delusional patients and their tendency to form new words. Forbes Winslow reported under "morbid phenomena of speech" patients with dysarthria, aphasia, obsessional utterances, mutism, and thought disorder, such as:

> "the 20 year-old man who was seized with a kind of cramp in the muscles of his mouth, accompanied with a sense of tickling upon the surface of his body, as if ants were creeping over it. After having experienced an attack of giddiness and mental confusion, a remarkable alteration in his speech was observed. He articulated easily and fluently, but made use of strange words which nobody could understand. . . ." (Winslow, 1861, pp. 471–510)

Guislain was even clearer in his definition of *d'incohérence des idées:*

> "the madman responds with a series of disconnected phrases and words. The deficit seems to be in *the mechanism that forms and combines words* before these are confided to the tongue. There is nothing wrong with this latter muscle for there is no deviation or the least difficulty in its movements. The disturbance is higher, it is in the brain . . . it is uncommon to observe incoherence of ideas which are not accompanied by delusions . . . Thus, the patient I have just shown believed he was the emperor." (p. 316, Guislain, 1852, my italics)

Guislain proposed a syndromatic view: "incoherence of ideas can be seen in extreme old age, after stroke, after delusional mania, and in the defect state of mania" (p. 317). By 'mania', Guislain meant delusional insanity (mainly schizophrenia-like states) rather than mania in the current sense of the term. As an explanation for this *obscuration des facultés intellectuelles*, Guislain suggested a mechanism of 'moral pain' (Guislain, 1852, vol. 2, pp. 148–149).

Griesinger (1861), in turn, divided the 'anomalies of thought' into 'formal deviations' (*formale Abweichungen*) and 'false contents' (*falscher Inhalt der Gedanken* – i.e. delusions and obsessions). He believed that "too rapid succession of the ideas, extreme slowness in the course of thought, or disorder of the feelings accompanying them, might excite and promote morbid ideas" (Griesinger, 1861, p. 67). There also was "incoherence of thought and speech [*verwirrte Incohärenz im Denken und Reden*], corresponding to projections of the thoughts and of the emotions, as anger," and "still another which proceeds from incomplete abolition and deep destruction of the mental processes". Griesinger also suggested a mechanism for these disorders, perhaps the first theory of formal thought disorder in the history of psychiatry:

> "it appears that the incoherence depends on the fact that the perceptions are called forth, not only according to their (similar or contrasting) contents, but *specially according to external similarity of sounds in the words. Perhaps deficient reciprocal action of the two halves of the brain* may have some influence in producing incoherence." (Griesinger, 1861, p. 68, my italics)

Griesinger's view on the psychopathology of thought disorder originated in the model of information processing developed by Herbart (De Garmo, 1896; Fritzsch, 1932; Ackerknecht, 1965; Wahrig-Schmidt, 1965) and in Wigan's ideas on the 'double brain' (Wigan, 1844).

Lastly, mention should be made of the work of Jules Falret, who in his "Aphasie, aphémie et alalie" suggested for the first time a separation between the neurological and psychiatric disorders of language. Thus, commenting upon Jaccoud's classification of 'alalia', he wrote:

"I believe that it is convenient to limit the meaning of this word . . . on the one hand there are the disorders of language due to lesions of the organs involved in the articulation of sound, and on the other those resulting from general disorders of intellect or various forms of mental disorder. In this latter case, language disorders are secondary to a general affection of the intellectual functions and deserve separate description." (Falret, 1866, p. 610)

Although not quoting Falret by name, Wernicke (1874, p. 70) did echo this distinction between neurological and psychiatric disorders of language. Surprisingly, Freud (1953) did not discuss the psychiatric disorders of language in his 1891 monograph on aphasia, in spite of the fact that he tried to develop a more dynamic view of these disorders.

However, during the latter part of the century, questions on the meaning and nature of the psychiatric disorders of language were obscured by the debate on aphasia and brain localisation. The old notion of a directive centre was also challenged, particularly by the 'holistic' account put forward by Hughlings Jackson (see Head, 1915, and below). Likewise, the renaissance of the associationistic or 'switchboard' paradigm affected the thinking of the new generation of alienists. For example, the young Gilbert Ballet (1886) succumbed to that approach in his first book, entitled *Le Langage Intérieur et les Diverses Formes de l'Aphasie*. Overoptimistically, Ballet claimed that the problem of language had been almost resolved, and subsumed all forms of language disturbance under the same neurological model. Very different was to be Séglas's book, six years later.

Jackson's views on thought and language

Jackson's complex ideas on language and its disturbances are only tangentially relevant to the history of thought disorder (Riese, 1955, 1965). Jackson:

(a) favoured a 'semantic' as opposed to a 'mechanistic' definition of speech
(b) attacked the concept of a 'faculty' of language (central to the French debate)
(c) interpreted the afflictions of speech in terms of a hierarchical model (as he had done in the case of epilepsy and stroke)
(d) borrowed from Spencer the view that there were both intellectual and emotional modes of expression (López Piñero, 1973; Dewhurst, 1982).

Jackson (1932, pp. 159–160) wrote:

"to speak is not only to utter words, it is to propositionise. A proposition is such a relation of words that it makes one new meaning . . . [therefore] loss of speech is the loss of power to propositionise."

He opposed the view that language is just the result of mechanical associations of words and that what puts the words together into propositions is a special faculty of language. On this, he remained loyal to Locke and the empiricist tradition; his solution, however, was not altogether clear, for he believed that, apart from words, there was nothing else localised in the brain:

"we do not mean by using the popular term power, that the speechless man has lost any 'faculty' of speech or propositioning; he has lost those words which serve in speech, the nervous arrangements for them being destroyed. There is no 'faculty' or 'power' of speech apart from words revived or revivable, any more than there is a faculty of 'co-ordination' of movements apart from movements represented in particular ways." (Jackson, 1932, p. 160)

Jackson's view that the afflictions of speech resulted from 'dissolution' led him to postulate both 'negative' and 'positive' components. Automatic speech and other 'release' or positive phenomena were not the meaningless results of a brain lesion, but the expression of a healthy site: hence the information contained therein was expected to be organised according to specific rules. It has been rightly suggested that this notion was important to the development of Freud's views on language, the unconscious, and of the view that thought disorder was the expression of an unconscious mentation (Fullinwider, 1983).

Séglas and his book

Louis Jules Ernest Séglas's life was exactly coterminous with Freud's, both having been born in May of 1856, and died in 1939. Séglas trained at the Bicêtre and Salpêtrière hospitals, and excelled in the area of descriptive psychopathology (see, for example, his magnificent "Séméiologie des affections mentales" (Séglas, 1903)). His book on *Des Troubles du Langage chez les Aliénés* was based on lectures delivered for three years at Salpêtrière and appeared in a medical series edited by Charcot (who was to die a year later) (Séglas, 1892). A first-class clinician and close friend of Chaslin, he is said to have disliked the limelight.

Séglas started with the basic point that, although the diagnosis of mental illness is carried out by the identification of symptoms such as delusions, hallucinations, mood disorder, and so on, the process itself was mediated by language and by the analysis of linguistic expressions and gestures. He divided disorders of language in those affecting speech, writing, or mimicry. The first group comprised disorders due to pathology of thought (*dyslogies*) (although Andreasen (1982, p. 297) has written: "Dyslogia is a *new term* [my italics], but one which derives from familiar roots"), of language (*dysphasies*), and of speech (*dyslalies*).

According to whether tempo, form, syntax, or content of language was disordered, four types of dyslogia could be identified. *Tempo* could be increased (e.g. *logorrhée, polyphrasie de Kussmaül, fuite des idées, langage elliptique, lalomanie*) or decreased; in the latter case it was characterised by retardation and could end up in *mutisme vésanique*. Alterations in the *form* of language included changes in timbre, imitations of animal sounds, obscene or pompous terminology, verbigeration (as per Kahlbaum), and plaintiveness. Changes in *syntax* included referring to the self as a third person, using clumsy turns of phrase, or disintegration of word construction. Changes in *content* comprised fixation on certain themes (*paralogie thématique*), stereotypies, and neologisms, which could be passive (resulting from automatic processes) or active (when the patient voluntarily invented new terms). Séglas included a lengthy discussion on neologisms (see pp. 46–66). The only important work on this topic before Séglas had been Bartels (1888), and since then it has been Cenac (1925) and Bobon (1952).

Séglas also studied dyslogia resulting from emotional and reflex language disturbance. The former included, for example, flat, monotonous or vivacious language, and language with cadence (in keeping with the subject's mood); the latter might be triggered by certain stimuli and included echolalia (and what Robertson in Britain called 'automatic speech').

Finally, disturbances of mimicry were divided according to whether they were related or unrelated to thought disorder; the former including changes in expression, gestural mannerisms, and so on.

The dysphasias, in turn, could be organic and functional; the latter group including transient verbal amnesias, verbal hallucinations, and verbal impulsions.

Dyslalias resulted from congenital causes, bad learning, neurological disease, and spasmodic neuroses.

Verbigerations were divided by Séglas into oral (considered as a disorder of the form of speech without actual pathology of language, p. 38) and written forms (p.230):

"When the problem is due to a disorder of thought, the function of language rests intact. In this case the distortion of speech will betray a primary disorder of intellect." (p. 16)

It is difficult to imagine a more detailed description of thought disorder and cognate states. For reasons which are unclear, recent authors have played down (e.g. Pinard & Lecours, 1983) or ignored his contribution altogether (Boyer, 1981).

Séglas refrained from quoting his theoretical sources, and ventured little in the way of explanatory hypotheses. It is clear, however, that he considered the disorders of language as 'symptoms' which could be present in various mental disorders (Lanteri-Laura & Del Pistoia, 1980). Only in a few cases did he suggest that there might be an association between a symptom and a particular disease.

Masselon and 'thought disorder'

A disciple of Sérieux, Masselon was 28 years old when he published his empirical study on the psychology of dementia praecox (Masselon, 1905). Against strong French opposition to the Kraepelinian concept, Masselon evaluated some psychological functions and psychiatric symptoms of 13 subjects suffering from dementia praecox. The former included attention (by means of Ribot's model), reaction time both simple and choice (using Phillips' chronometric paradigm), memory (both for recent and remote events), mood, and motor behaviour. Thought disorder, in turn, was assessed as coordination of ideas and intellectual weakness and deterioration.

Masselon found that his subjects showed marked impairment of attention, particularly what he called 'voluntary' attention; they were found to be easily distractible, and perceptually bound. Both reaction times were prolonged, particularly choice reaction time. Memory was affected, as was mood, all patients showing apathy, flatness, and aboulia. Thought processes were also impaired, the commonest disorder involving judgement and synthesis of thought. Subjects showed fixation on few themes, stereotypies, puerility, echolalia, tics of language, and marked reduction in their capacity to monitor the environment.

Masselon concluded that '*démence précoce*' was a disease that caused a primary impairment of the active faculties of the mind. Apathy, aboulia, and loss of intellectual power constituted the central triad of the disease. These impairments caused 'secondary affective disturbance' (pp. 259–265).

Views on thought disorder after Masselon

Up to this period, associationism had governed the understanding of thought disorder. Kraepelin's views (based on Wundtian psychology) were no exception, and among the pathognomonic 'psychic symptoms' of dementia praecox, he listed typical forms such as disorder of judgement, stereotypies, incoherence of the train of thought, derailments in linguistic expression, paraphasias, neologisms, akataphasia (inability to find the appropriate expression for a thought), impairment in the construction of sentences, and speaking past the subject (Kraepelin, 1919).

Bleuler, with the help of the psychologist Gustav Jung, also considered thought disorder as central to 'schizophrenia', the term he created to replace dementia praecox (Berrios, 1987). As far as mechanisms for these disorders were concerned, Bleuler remained loyal to the old associationist theory.

Jung's work (1972) on the psychology of dementia praecox was published four years before Bleuler's (1911).

Jung's monograph has three parts: a historical review of the literature, a comparison of dementia praecox and hysteria, and a long report of the case of a 62-year-old woman (first admitted aged 42) with a putative diagnosis of dementia praecox. The review mainly dealt with the work of Gross (1904), Stransky (1904), Weygandt (1904, 1907), and Janet (1903), and, not surprisingly, Masselon (1905). Jung wrote of the latter: "In Masselon's work we find an assortment of views which he feels all go back to the one root, but he cannot find this root without obscuring his work" (p. 11).

Jung concluded that earlier results "converged towards the same goal . . . the idea of quite central disturbance which is called by various names: apperceptive deterioration (Weygandt); dissociation, *abaissement du niveau mental* (Masselon, Janet); disintegration of consciousness (Gross); disintegration of personality (Neisser *et al*)" (p. 37). Jung agreed that, as far as thought disorder was concerned, there was a disturbance of associations, but he complained that little was known as to how to separate abnormal from normal or unimpaired thinking: "In dementia praecox, where as a matter of fact countless normal associations still exist, we must expect that until we get to know the very delicate processes which are really specific of the disease the laws of the normal psyche will long continue to play their part" (p. 7).

Jung believed that similar pathological processes operated in hysteria and dementia praecox:

> "in dementia praecox, too, we find one or more complexes which have become permanently fixed and could not, therefore, be overcome. But whereas in persons predisposed to hysteria there is an unmistakable causal connection between the complexes and the illness, in dementia praecox it is not at all clear whether the complex caused or precipitated the illness." (p. 97)

The crucial difference between the two, Jung thought, was the presence in dementia praecox of "hypothetical X, a metabolic toxin, and its effect on the psyche" (p. 98).

In schizophrenia, according to Bleuler, the

> "associations lose their continuity. Of the thousands of associative threads which guide our thinking, this disease seems to interrupt, quite haphazardly, sometimes such single threads, sometimes a whole group, and sometimes even large segments of them. In this way, thinking becomes illogical and often bizarre." (Bleuler, 1911, p. 10)

Bleuler tried to explain subsymptoms as combinations and permutations of such disconnections.

The views of Jung and Bleuler, as those of Janet, Berze and Rignano, reflect a move away from neurological explanations. For example, Berze (1914) proposed (like Janet) an 'energetist' hypothesis, which he called 'primary insufficiency'; and Rignano (1922, pp. 238–244) supported a view of thought disorder based on a reduction of energy and in changes in the affective sphere.

Few continued with the organicist line; thus Kleist (1930) wrote:

"I was able to isolate in 1914, from the many varieties of confused speech which one sees in that condition, several particular disturbances which could be regarded as based on cerebral pathology. In doing so I confirmed Kraepelin's hypothesis that some schizophrenic disorders of speech depend, like similar phenomena that are found in dream speech, on functional disturbances in the temporal speech area."

Yet others, like Jaspers, steered a middle course: speech disorders in the psychoses

"include certain verbal performances which at present cannot be explained in terms of neurological mechanisms; nor can they be simply understood as a form of expression or as the communication of abnormal psychic contents. We have to deal with a territory of interest to both sides." (Jaspers, 1963, p. 191)

The return of the holistic approach

After the First World War, the stage was set for a major challenge to associationism and localisationism (Lanteri-Laura, 1984). Born in different quarters, these ideas were all inspired by evolutionary theory. Some, following Jackson's view, proposed a return to 'holistic' approaches such as Henry Head's evolutionary neurophysiology (Piéron, 1927) or Lashley's (1963) notion of 'equipotentiality' (in brain localisation), or von Monakow's hierarchical view (in psychiatry) (von Monakow & Mourgue, 1928), or Koehler's (Peterman, 1932) and Koffka's (1928) Gestalt paradigms (in psychology).

Others developed evolutionary models based on imaginary differences between the mind or 'mentality' of 'primitive' races and that of civilised man (Lévy-Bruhl, 1928; Allier, 1929; Lévy-Valensi, 1934), thereby encouraging the view that thought processes in the insane were like those of primitive man (Blondel, 1914). The notion of mentality did not go unchallenged; for example, Leroy (1927) expressed surprise at Jung's uncritical acceptance of the notion of pre-logical mentality. More recently, Lloyd (1990) has attacked the general concept of mentality.

The state of theory at this time is well reflected in the comment by Kasanin & Lewis:

"After World War I, formal investigations in the field of schizophrenic thinking were stopped for almost two decades because of the extreme interest of the psychiatrist in the dynamic aspects of psychiatry as expressed in the teaching of Meyer, Freud, Jung and others. These investigators pointed out that schizophrenic speech utterances have a definite meaning and content even though they may be quite distorted and incomprehensible to the observer." (Kasanin & Lewis, 1944, p. 2) (for excellent reviews of the history of schizophrenic language see Piro, 1967; Reed, 1970)

Kurt Goldstein explored schizophrenic thinking from the point of view of Gestalt psychology, and compared it with thinking processes in brain-damaged subjects. In both groups there was a fundamental change in the boundaries between figure and background (i.e. a disappearance of the normal boundaries between the ego and the world). Although both organic and schizophrenic subjects showed 'concrete' thinking, the latter's performance showed intrusions related to delusional and other psychotic material (Goldstein, 1944; see also Payne *et al*, 1959).

Schilder took a similar view. In a paper on the psychology of general paralysis, he dealt with thought disorder from a Gestalt viewpoint; patients with thought disorder used:

"inexpedient methods in registration, elaboration and reproduction. The necessary anticipations and the integration of parts into wholes do not take place. The whole-apperceptions that do come about are not sufficiently structured. In the process of apperception concepts and situations are [freely] replaced by co-ordinate or superordinate concepts." (Schilder, 1930; on apperception see Lange, 1900)

Von Domarus published his classic paper on schizophrenic thinking in 1927 (Von Domarus, 1927). Later on, and influenced by Vygotsky, he suggested that schizophrenic patients differed from the normal in that they were 'paralogical', that is, they did not require 'identity of all predicates' to state that two objects were identical: they might say that an orange and a house were the same simply because both shared one attribute (say the colour orange). On occasions, the predicate may be something which was not even apparent to the observer (e.g. that both were facing north). Von Domarus generalised from very few patients, and used no controls in his clinical analysis (Von Domarus, 1944) (on Vygotsky see Wertsch, 1985).

Conclusions

From this short history of the concept of thought disorder, it can be concluded that this 'symptom' refers to a heterogeneous group of behaviours which, during the last 100 years, have been given uniformity and unity by the

Procrustean device of reinterpreting them according to successive theories of thinking. During the time of association theory, emphasis was given to the connection of ideas (Billod, 1861), and the assumption was made that language and thought were so closely associated that disturbances of the one necessarily showed in the other. This theory inspired the original work on 'thought disorder' by Griesinger, Séglas, and Masselon. Kraepelin, Jung and Bleuler add little to these early insights, their contribution being limited to claiming that such a symptom was primary to the diagnosis of schizophrenia. With the decline of associationism, and the growth of holistic psychologies and evolutionary theory, thinking was redefined in terms of the recognition of wholes and of concept-making. This led to new ways of describing thought disorder, which then became a disturbance of concept formation (Kasanin & Haufmann, 1938) due to some putative breakdown in logical rules.

The main lesson to be drawn from this historical account is that 'thought disorder' is a construct, a 'symptom' which remains parasitical upon theories of thinking. This means that, whether formulated in terms of association theory or of information processing, attentional, or computational models, or indeed considered as a speech disorder (Chaika, 1982), the actual 'behaviour' involved (i.e. talking weird or nonsense) is unlikely to be localisable in the brain in the way in which other symptoms (e.g. hallucination) might be.

This chapter has focused on the contribution of some German and French alienists, who, although less well known than Kussmaul, Jaccoud, Charcot or Jackson, were equally important to the shaping of modern views.

By the end of the 19th century, the vague category 'language and speech disorder' had become that of formal thought disorder (and considered a pathognomonic feature of dementia praecox). Masselon offered the first important empirical study of this phenomenon (before Kraepelin and Bleuler).

The work of Séglas is of particular relevance in this context, and a detailed account has been offered of his ideas. Since his time, and caught between the psychological and organic horns of the aetiological dilemma, the mechanisms underlying the disorders of language in psychiatry have remained obscure; indeed, their clinical status has not yet been fully elucidated.

References

ACKERKNECHT, E. H. (1965) Preface. In *Mental Pathology and Therapeutics* (W. Griesinger). New York: Hafner.

ALLIER, R. (1929) *The Mind of the Savage*. London: Bell.

ANDREASEN, N. C. (1982) Should the term "thought disorder" be revised? *Comprehensive Psychiatry*, **23**, 291–299.

BAILLARGER, J. (1865) De l'aphasie au point de vue psychologique. In *Recherches sur les Maladies Mentales* (Idem, 1890), pp. 584–601. Paris: Masson.

BALLET, G. (1886) *Le Langage Intérieur et les Diverses Formes de l'Aphasie.* Paris: Alcan.
BARTELS, I. (1884). Über Wortneubildung bei Geisteskranken. *Allgemeine Zeitschrift für Psychiatrie,* **45**, 598–601.
BENSON, D. F. (1973) Psychiatric aspects of aphasia. *British Journal of Psychiatry,* **123**, 555–566.
BERRIOS, G. E. (1987) Introduction to Bleuler's work. In *The Origins of Modern Psychiatry* (ed. C. Thompson), pp. 200–209. Chichester: Wiley.
BERZE, J. (1914) *Die Primäre Insuffizienz der psychischen Aktivität.* Leipzig: Deuticke.
BILLOD, E. (1861) De la lésion de l'association des idées. *Annales Médico-Psychologiques,* **18**, 540–552.
BLAKEY, R. (1850) *History of the Philosophy of Mind, Vol. 1,* pp. 375–410. London: Longman, Brown, Green & Longman.
BLEULER, E. (1911) *Dementia Praecox.* Leipzig: Franz Deuticke.
BLONDEL, CH. (1914) *La Conscience Morbide. Essai de Psycho-Pathologie Générale.* Paris: Alcan.
BOBON, J. (1952) *Introduction Historique à l'Étude des Néologismes et des Glossolalies en Psychopathologie.* Paris: Masson.
BOUILLAUD, J. B. (1825) Recherches cliniques propres à démontrer que la perte de la parole correspond à la lésion des lobules antérieurs du cerveau, et à confirmer l'opinion de M. Gall, sur le siège de l'organe du langage articulé. *Archives Générales de Médecine,* **8**, 25–45.
BOYER, P. (1981) *Les Troubles du Langage en Psychiatrie.* Paris: Presses Universitaires de France.
BROOKS, G. P. (1976) The faculty psychology of Thomas Reid. *Journal of the History of the Behavioral Sciences,* **12**, 65–77.
BUJOSA, F. (1980) Reconsideraciones sobre la historia de la afasia. In *Medicina e Historia* (eds A. Albarracín, J. M. López-Piñero & L. S. Granjel) pp. 305–320. Madrid: Editorial de la Universidad Complutense.
CASSIRER, E. (1929) La pathologie de la conscience symbolique. *Journal de Psychologie Normale et Pathologique,* **26**, 625–709.
CENAC, M. (1925) *De Certains Langages Créés par les Aliénés: Contribution à l'Etude des 'Glossolalies'.* Thèse de Médicine, Paris.
CHAIKA, E. (1982) Thought disorder or speech disorder in schizophrenia. *Schizophrenia Bulletin,* **8**, 587–591.
CLAPARÈDE, É. (1903) *L'Association des Idées.* Paris: Doin.
COMBE, G. (1873) *Elements of Phrenology* (10th edn). Edinburgh: MacLachlan & Stewart.
CRITCHLEY, M. (1964) The neurology of psychotic speech. *British Journal of Psychiatry,* **110**, 353–364.
DAUZAT, A. (1912) *La Philosophie du Langage.* Paris: Flammarion.
DE GARMO, C. (1896) *Herbart and the Herbartians.* New York: Scribner.
DEWHURST, K. (1982) *Hughlings Jackson on Psychiatry.* Oxford: Sandford.
FALRET, J. (1866) Aphasie, aphémie, alalie. In *Dictionnaire Encyclopédique des Sciences Médicales, Vol. 5* (eds A. Dechambre & L. Lereboullet), pp. 605–644. Paris: Masson.
FOURNIER-PESCAY, T. & BÉGIN, M. (1821) Parole. In Panckouke's *Dictionaire des Sciences Médicales, Vol. 39,* (ed. Panckouke), pp. 306–354.
FREUD, S. (1953) *On Aphasia* (translation of E. Stengel). London: Imago. (Original German edition, 1891.)
FRITZSCH, T. (1932) *Juan Federico Herbart.* Barcelona: Labor.
FULLINWIDER, S. P. (1983) Sigmund Freud, John Hughlings Jackson, and speech. *Journal of the History of Ideas,* **44**, 151–158.
GARNIER, A. (1852) *Traité des Facultés de l'Ame, Vol. 3.* Paris: Hachette.
GOLDSTEIN, K. (1944) Methodological approach to the study of schizophrenic thought disorder. In *Language and Thought in Schizophrena* (eds J. S. Kasanin & N. D. C. Lewis), pp. 17–40. New York: Norton.
GRIESINGER, W. (1861) *Die Pathologie und Therapie der psychischen Krankheiten* (2nd edn). Stuttgart: Krabbe.
GROSS, O. (1904) Dementia sejunctiva. *Neurologisches Centralblatt,* **23**, 1144–1146.
GUISLAIN, J. (1852) *Leçons Orales sur les Phrénopathies, Vol. 1.* Gand: Hebbelnyck.
HAMILTON, M. (ed.) (1974) *Fish's Clinical Psychopathology.* Bristol: Wright.
HEAD, H. (1915) Hughlings Jackson on aphasia. *Brain,* **38**, 1–190.

HÉCAEN, H. & DUBOIS, J. (1969) *La Naissance de la Neuropsychologie du Langage.* Paris: Flammarion.
HILGARD, E. R. (1980) The trilogy of mind: cognition, affection, and conation. *Journal of the History of the Behavioral Sciences,* **16,** 107–117.
HUGO, V. (1856) *Contemplations,* I, viii, 1.
IGGERS, G. G. (1973) Historicism. In *Dictionary of the History of Ideas Vol. 2* (ed. P. P. Wiener), pp. 456–464. New York: Scribner.
JACKSON, J. H. (1932) *Selected Writings of John Hughlings Jackson.* London: Hodder & Stoughton.
JANET, P. (1903) *Les Obsessions et la Psychasthénie.* Paris: Alcan.
JASPERS, K. (1963) *General Psychopathology* (1st edn, 1913). Manchester: Manchester University Press.
JOURNAL OF MENTAL SCIENCE (1892) Review. *Journal of Mental Science,* **38,** 594–596.
JULIARD, P. (1970) *Philosophies of Language in Eighteenth Century France.* The Hague: Mouton.
JUNG, C. G. (1972) *The Psychology of Dementia Praecox.* In *The Collected Works, Vol. 3* (1st edn, 1904). London: Routledge & Kegan Paul.
KASANIN, J. & HAUFMANN, E. (1938) Disturbances in concept formation in schizophrenia. *Archives of Neurology and Psychiatry,* **40,** 1276–1282.
—— & LEWIS, N. C. D. (eds) (1944) *Language and Thought in Schizophrenia.* New York: W. W. Norton.
KIRKLAND, T. (1792) *A Commentary on Apoplectic and Paralytic Affections.* London: Dawson.
KLEIST, K. (1930) Zur hirnpathologischen Auffassung der schizophrenen Grundstörungen. Die alogische Denkstörung. *Schweizer Archiv für Neurologie und Psychiatrie,* **26,** 99–102.
—— (1960) Schizophrenic symptoms and cerebral pathology. *Journal of Mental Science,* **106,** 246–255.
KNOLL, E. (1982) The science of language and the evolution of mind: Max Müller's quarrel with Darwinism. *Journal of the History of the Behavioral Sciences,* **22,** 3–22.
KOERNER, E. F. K. (1982) *Ferdinand de Saussure.* Madrid: Gredos.
KOFFKA, K. (1928) *The Growth of the Mind* (2nd edn). London: Kegan Paul.
KRAEPELIN, E. (1919) *Dementia Praecox and Paraphrenia* (trans. R. M. Barclay & G. M. Robertson). Edinburgh: E. & S. Livingstone.
LANDRE-BEAUVAIS, A. J. (1813) *Séméiotique, ou Traité des Signes de Maladies.* Paris: Brosson.
LANGE, K. (1900) *Apperception.* Boston: Heath.
LANTERI-LAURA, G. (1984) Les localisations imaginaires. *L'Evolution Psychiatrique,* **49,** 379–402.
—— & DEL PISTOIA, L. (1980) Diversité clinique et unité physio-psychopathologique des altérations du langage. *L'Evolution Psychiatrique,* **45,** 225–252.
LASHLEY, K. S. (1963) *Brain Mechanisms and Intelligence* (1st edn, 1929). New York: Dover.
LEROY, M. (1969) *Las Grandes Corrientes de la Linguistica.* México City: Fondo de Cultura Económica.
LEROY, O. (1927) *La Raison Primitive. Essai de Réfutation de la Théorie du Prélogisme.* Paris: Alcan.
LÉVY-BRUHL, L. (1928) *Les Fonctions Mentales dans les Sociétés Inférieures* (1st edn, 1910). Paris: Alcan.
LÉVY-VALENSI, J. (1934) Mentalité primitive et psychopathologie. *Annales Médico-Psychologiques,* **92,** 676–701.
LLOYD, G. E. R. (1990) *Demystifying Mentalities.* Cambridge: Cambridge University Press.
LÓPEZ PIÑERO, J. M. (1973) *John Hughlings Jackson (1835–1911).* Madrid: Moneda.
LORDAT, J. (1843) Analyse de la parole pour servir à la théorie de divers cas d'alalie et de paralalie (de mutisme et d'imperfection du parler) que les nosologistes ont mal connus. *Journal de la Société de Médecine Pratique de Montpellier,* **7,** 333–353.
MACEVOY, H. J. (1900) Review. *Journal of Mental Science,* **46,** 542–543.
MARX, O. (1966) Aphasia studies and language theory in the 19th century. *Bulletin of the History of Medicine,* **40,** 328–349.
MASSELON, R. (1905) *Psychologie des Déments Précoces.* Thèse pour le Doctorat en Médecine. Paris: L. Boyer.
MONAKOW, C. & MOURGUE, R. (1928) *Introduction Biologique à l'Etude de la Neurologie et de la Psychopathologie.* Paris: Alcan.
MONCALM, M. (1900) *En l'Origine de la Pensée et de la Parole.* Paris: Alcan.
MOUTIER, F. (1908) *L'Aphasie de Broca.* Paris: Steinheil.

MÜLLER, M. (1882) *Lectures on the Science of Language, Vol. 1.* London: Longmans, Green.
O'NEILL, Y. V. (1980) *Speech and Speech Disorders in Western Thought Before 1600.* London: Greenwood Press.
PAULHAN, F. (1889) *L'Activité Mentale et les Eléments de l'Esprit.* Paris: Alcan.
PAYNE, R. W., MATTUSSEK, P. & GEORGE, E. I. (1959) An experimental study of schizophrenic thought disorder. *Journal of Mental Science*, **105**, 627-652.
PETERMAN, B. (1932) *The Gestalt Theory and the Problem of Configuration.* London: Kegan Paul.
PIÉRON, H. (1927) *Thought and the Brain.* London: Kegan Paul, Trench, Trubner.
PINARD, G. & LECOURS, A. R. (1983) The language of psychotics and neurotics. In *Aphasiology* (eds A. R. Lecours, F. L'Hermitte & B. Bryans), pp. 313-335. London: Baillière.
PIROS, S. (1967) *Il Linguaggio Schizofrenico.* Milan: Giangiacomo Feltrinelli.
PORTER, N. (1868) *The Human Intellect.* New York: Scribner.
RAUB, C. Q. (1988) Robert Chambers and William Whewell: a nineteenth century debate over the origin of language. *Journal of the History of Ideas*, **49**, 287-300.
REED, J. L. (1970) Schizophrenic thought disorder: a review and hypothesis. *Comprehensive Psychiatry*, **11**, 403-432.
RIESE, W. (1955) Hughlings Jackson's doctrine of aphasia and its significance today. *Journal of Nervous and Mental Disease*, **122**, 1-13.
—— (1965) The sources of Hughlings Jackson's view on aphasia. *Brain*, **88**, 811-822.
RIGNANO, E. (1922) *Psicología del Razonamiento* (1st Italian edn 1920). Madrid: Calpe.
ROCKEY, D. (1980) *Speech Disorders in Nineteenth Century Britain.* London: Croom Helm.
SCHILDER, P. (1930) *Studien zur Psychologie und Symptomatologie der progressiven Paralyse.* Berlin: Karger.
SÉGLAS, J. (1892) *Des Troubles du Langage chez les Aliénés.* Paris: J. Rueff.
—— (1903) Séméiologie des affections mentales. In *Traité de Pathologie Mentale* (ed. G. Ballet), pp. 74-270. Paris: Octave Doin.
SNELL, L. (1852) Über die veränderte Sprechweise und die Bildung neurer Worte und Ausdrucke in Wahnsinn. *Allgemeine Zeitschrift für Psychiatrie*, **9**, 11-23.
SOCIÉTÉ DE LINGUISTIQUE DE PARIS (1868) *Mémoires de la Société de Linguistique de Paris*, **1**, 3.
SPOERL, H. D. (1936) Faculties versus traits: Galls's solution. *Character and Personality*, **4**, 216-231.
SPURZHEIM, G. (1826) *Phrenology.* London: Treuttel.
STAROBINSKI, J. (1974) The role of language in psychiatric treatment in the French Romantic Age. *Psychological Medicine*, **4**, 360-363.
STRANSKY, E. (1904) Zur Auffassung gewisser Symptome der Dementia praecox. *Neurologisches Centralblatt*, **23**, 1137-1143.
TAINE, H. (1871) *On Intelligence.* London: Reeve.
VON DOMARUS, E. (1927) Zur Theories des schizophrenen Denkens. *Zeitschrift für Neurologie und Psychiatrie*, **108**, 703-714.
—— (1944) The specific laws of logic in schizophrenia. In *Language and Thought in Schizophrenia* (eds J. S. Kasanin & N. D. C. Lewis), pp. 104-114. New York: W. W. Norton.
WAHRIG-SCHMIDT, B. (1965) *Der junge Wilhelm Griesinger im Spannusgsfeld zwischen Philosophie und Physiologie.* Tübingen: Gunter Narr.
WARREN, H. C. (1921) *History of the Association Psychology.* New York: Scribner.
WERNICKE, C. (1874) *Der Aphasische Symptomencomplex.* Breslau: Max Cohn & Weigert.
WERTSCH, J. V. (1985) *Vigotsky and the Social Formation of Mind.* Cambridge, Mass.: Harvard University Press.
WEYGANDT, W. (1904) Alte Dementia praecox. *Neurologisches Centralblatt*, **23**, 613-617.
—— (1907) Kritische Bemerkungen zur Psychologie der Dementia praecox. *Monatsschrift für Psychiatrie und Neurologie*, **22**, 289-301.
WIGAN, A. L. (1844) *The Duality of the Mind.* London: Longman, Brown, Green & Longman.
WINSLOW, F. (1861) *On Obscure Diseases of the Brain and Disorders of the Mind* (2nd edn). London: John W. Davies.

3 Analysis of language: terminology and techniques

DAVID NEWBY

That there are oddities in the language produced by many patients with psychiatric disorder seems indisputable. Indeed, particularly with regard to the psychotic disorders, peculiar speech or communication is often one of the most tangible markers that there is something wrong. A prodigious amount of research effort has gone into attempting to understand just what is the nature and cause of the language disruption – if we can understand that, we may gain insights into the nature of the disorder itself.

Sadly, really worthwhile insights have been few and far between. In the last two or three decades, however, there has arisen a fruitful interchange of ideas between psychiatrists and experts in the field of language itself – linguists and psycholinguists. As such, it may be said that an 'interface' discipline has grown up, with contrasting models and ways of thinking being brought together to understand a common problem. Psychiatrists and psychologists probably have much to learn from linguists and psycholinguists in understanding the 'ramblings' of their patients, but it should not be forgotten that extremely valuable insights may be gained into the structure and function of language itself if we can understand more of what goes wrong in the 'thought-disordered' patient.

This chapter provides an overview of some terms and concepts from linguistics that will probably be unfamiliar to the general psychiatrist, in the hope that this will facilitate understanding of some of the advances referred to in other parts of the book. En route, some aspects of the basic relationship between thought and language are considered.

Basic definitions

The idea of 'language' itself has taxed generations of thinkers who have struggled to provide a comprehensive and yet still comprehensible definition.

A plethora of attempts has been offered, with wide or narrow focus according to circumstance. Some look towards the formal, structural qualities of language only; some embrace the wide range of functions that the structural system of language enables (e.g. imparting information, declaring a feeling, influencing the action of others, facilitating propositional thought). Some restrict themselves to human language systems; some encompass the communicatory conventions that animals may use (e.g. the 'dance' of bees, which codes in a highly formalised way the direction and size of a food source).

Crystal (1987, p. 396) cites a collection of definitions, which include the following:

> "The systematic, conventional use of sounds, signs or written symbols in a human society for communication and self-expression." (Crystal, 1987)
>
> "Audible, articulate, meaningful sound as produced by the action of the vocal organs." (*Webster's Third New International Dictionary*, 1961)
>
> "A set (finite or infinite) of sentences, each finite in length and constructed out of a finite set of elements." (Chomsky, 1957)

These vary in descriptive power, and seem to tap into different aspects of what we understand to be language, but none alone seems to capture the essence of the concept. The lesson to be drawn is that – like many concepts in psychiatry – the use of the word 'language' will vary greatly according to the user, and it is as well to be clear how the term is being used when interpreting research.

Relationship between thought and language

If 'language' is difficult to define, 'thought' must be more so. One of the recurrent problems arising in the field of research into language disorders is the failure to recognise the potential distinctions between thought and language. This is exemplified by the use of the clinical concept of 'formal thought disorder' (FTD). Most clinicians are quite good at recognising it – the 'disjointed', apparently non-goal-directed communications most commonly seen in patients with an acute functional psychosis. What is seldom appreciated is that what is being observed is the patient's *speech*, and that this may not directly reflect the flow of their thoughts. Without having access to a thought-reading machine, we can never be entirely sure of the latter, and for the most part can only infer thoughts from their counterparts in speech.

In a review article, Maher (1972) gave an apt analogy illustrating this distinction between thought and speech:

"The model might be likened to a typist copying from a script before her. Her copy may appear to be distorted because the script is distorted although the communication channel of the typist's eye and hand are functioning correctly. Alternatively, the original script may be perfect, but the typist may be unskilled, making typing errors in the copy and thus distorting it. Finally, it is possible for an inefficient typist to add errors to an already incoherent script. Unfortunately, the psychopathologist can observe only the copy (language utterances): he cannot examine the script (the thought). In general most theorists concerned with schizophrenic language have accepted the first of the three alternatives, namely that a good typist is transcribing a deviant script. The patient is correctly reporting a set of disordered thoughts."

All too often, the uncritical assumption has been made that speech directly mirrors thought. There are other lines of evidence which challenge this assumption.

Firstly, is it possible to have meaningful thought without the structure of language? Subjectively, most of us are aware that for the most part we think in language terms – for example, "I think it must be tea-time, wonder what's in the 'fridge?" What about day dreams, however? We can think ourselves in a particular situation without necessarily formulating it in words. This seemingly natural impression has been borne out, for example, by a study by Furth (1961) in the US, who looked at the development of concept formation in groups of deaf compared with hearing children aged between 7 and 12 years. The view had long been held that deaf children would inherently be inferior in activities requiring use of abstract concepts because of their relative lack of exposure to language (which carries the structure and description of those abstract concepts). Furth used tests which required the recognition of concepts of *sameness*, *symmetry*, and *opposition*. Sameness is so elementary or primitive that deaf children appear to understand it very early on, irrespective of their lack of a word to describe it. There should be no difference between groups on this ability. At the other extreme, the concept of symmetry is not coded in language terms for hearing children below the age of about 12 years, so again there should be no differential advantage for them. For 'opposition', however, our language is full of dimensional opposites, such as hot–cold, good–bad, and long–short. Exposure to these should facilitate the learning of the concept, predicted Furth, and thus advantage the hearing child in this task.

The results confirmed this. There were no significant differences between the groups on sameness and symmetry tasks, only on the opposition task. Although neither group had a word for symmetry, there were a few hearing *and* deaf children who succeeded on that task. The authors concluded that language exposure did facilitate concept attainment for some tasks, but that understanding was not always dependent on access to linguistic codes.

Proceeding in the other direction, one might ask whether language can proceed without thought? Malinowski (1972) described so-called 'phatic communication', in which this does indeed occur – speaking without thinking. What this amounts to is the everyday conventional speech we often use just as a means of basic social interaction, often without giving it much thought. For instance "Lovely day, isn't it?" may be uttered without us having given any real consideration to the matter.

So, thought and language are clearly linked and interdependent, but care must be taken in assuming a direct link. Mindful of these observations, Chaika (1982) has advocated substituting the concept of speech disorder for that of thought disorder.

Does language shape thought?

Lack of space precludes a full discussion of this interesting question, but a good account may be found, for example, in Slobin (1979). The ideas of 'linguistic determinism' and 'linguistic relativity' were propounded by Edward Sapir, a linguist, and a pupil of his, Benjamin Whorf. In essence, they suggested that how we view the world, and the relationships we perceive between things, is crucially determined by the structure of the language we happen to speak. An oft-cited example is the diversity of words in the Inuit language for snow. There is a whole range of words for different types of snow – snow suitable for sledging on, hard snow, soft snow, and so on, thus coding for nuances in the different types that might not be immediately obvious to non-Inuit speakers. How the Inuit view their largely snow-bound environment is, it is suggested, predetermined by the range of words they have available. Other examples abound, including distinctions in different languages for how tense is coded, how number is described, and so on.

It seems unlikely that cognitive structures are *entirely* determined by linguistic structures. At the very least, however, the structure of our language must have an effect on how we see the world in terms of the concepts that come most readily to us – as in the Furth experiments described above. Psychiatrists more than most should be aware of this: classification of psychiatric disorders is a movable feast. Today it seems quite natural to say "That patient is *schizophrenic*". A hundred years ago, the specific linguistic structure to say that would not have existed. A hundred years from now, who is to say that that term will not seem a misguided way to view people with certain mental afflictions? How we view our patients is to some extent shaped by the language we have available to describe them.

It would seem, then, that there is a two-way interaction between thought and language, the one shaping the other, as in Fig. 3.1.

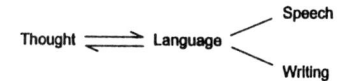

Fig. 3.1. The two-way interaction between thought and language

Levels of linguistic analysis

Having examined these basic relationships, it is appropriate to outline further how linguists and psycholinguists have sought to describe and understand language production and processing. Central to this is an understanding of the notion of *levels* of linguistic analysis. Take a simple sentence like:

(1) I find it rather cold in here.

In understanding such a sentence the listener will be (usually unconsciously) carrying out a number of different processes. At some point, the individual sound elements (the 'phonemes', or syllables) have to be recognised and parcelled into meaningful elements (ultimately 'words'). The structural relationships between the word elements (the grammar or syntax) must then be apprehended. For instance, in the example above, the listener must recognise that 'rather' and 'cold' are linked, the former modifying the latter. Then meaning must be mapped onto the individual elements and their relationships to produce finally some sense or meaning for the sentence as a whole. Presumably a mirror-image process occurs in the speaker producing such a sentence.

There are two important considerations here. Firstly, there is no universal agreement on how many levels should be set up to describe the process. Secondly, the above account implies a form of serial processing of language, in which one level has to be worked out before proceeding to the next level of complexity – a 'bottom-up' approach hypothesised, for example, by the linguist Leonard Bloomfield. This may be helpful in the academic understanding of language, but it should be remembered that actual processing in humans is unlikely to proceed in such a linear fashion.

As regards the number of levels, the simplest descriptions would recognise only two: *form* (the elements and structures), and *meaning*. This distinction can be seen as analagous to that between form and content in descriptive psychopathology. It is helpful, however, to subdivide the levels further, and the rest of this account follows the six-level model advocated in Crystal (1987) and illustrated in Fig. 3.2.

Phonetics and phonology

A 'phoneme' has been defined as "the smallest contrastive unit in the sound system of a language". An example would be the phonemes /b/ and /p/,

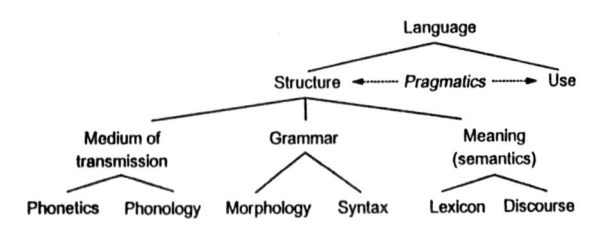

Fig. 3.2. Levels of linguistic/language analysis (from Crystal, 1987)

which make the differences between the words bat and pat. Phonology deals with how these units are amalgamated in relation to syntax.

Morphemes and morphology

At the next level of organisation, the 'morpheme' has been defined as "the smallest contrastive unit of grammar". Examples would be 'man', 'hit', the prefix 'de-' and the suffix '-tion'. Morphology is the study of how these units are structurally related, as for example in the word 'deglutition', where the morphemes 'de-' (down), '-gluti-' (swallowing) and '-tion' together make up 'the act of swallowing down'.

Grammar and syntax

To a greater or lesser extent, we are all familiar with the notion of grammar as taught in the school room. More mature psychiatrists may well have unwelcome recollections of arduous hours labouring over parts of speech, subjunctives, and various declensions. These are aspects of so-called traditional or prescriptive grammars, which are essentially static descriptions of acceptable word constructions in a particular language. To the linguist, 'grammar' has a much wider connotation, covering many aspects of the structures or patterns in language, and including constructs assumed to be common to many different languages. Again, however, there are differences in usage, with two quite distinct ways in which the term is used. Most commonly, grammar is viewed as just one aspect of language structure (Fig. 3.3a), in which case, grammar refers to the study of word order and patterns within a sentence. In a more general application, grammar is taken to subsume all aspects of sentence patterning and structure (Fig. 3.3b), in which case 'syntax' takes over the more specific connotation. For this reason, the two terms are interchangeable in different models of language.

Chomsky (1957) defined a grammar as "a device of some sort for producing the sentences of the language under analysis". Essentially, the task of any theoretical grammar is to describe a system or set of rules which can generate grammatical sentences and distinguish them from ungrammatical ones.

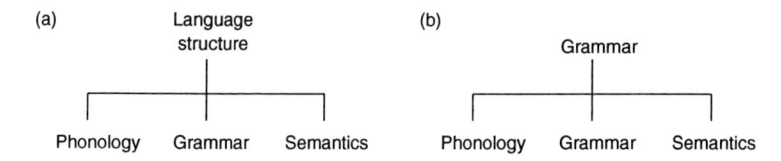

Fig. 3.3. Usages of 'grammar': (a) as one aspect of language structure; (b) as subsuming all aspects of sentence pattern and structure

For instance, given the two sentences:

(2) That car cost a lot of money.
(3) *A lot of money was cost by that car.

Most native speakers of English would instinctively recognise the second to be ungrammatical (* is conventionally used in linguistics to denote an unacceptable construction). A grammar must explain why (3) is unacceptable, despite the fact that it is clearly related to (2) – a passive transformation of it in fact.

Transformational or generative grammars

This topic could reasonably be described as having revolutionised much of the thinking in modern linguistics. Noam Chomsky has made the most important contributions here. Central to his work is the notion of 'deep structure'. This may be exemplified by another pair of sentences:

(4) The dog chased the rabbit.
(5) The rabbit was chased by the dog.

Sentence (4) involves an active sentence construction, and (5) is its directly related passive equivalent. Native speakers have no difficulty in recognising that, in spite of quite different surface appearances, the two sentences describe the same situation: they mean the same thing. To account for this, Chomsky posited that there was a single 'deep structure' underlying such sentences, and that a definable set of 'transformational rules' could be described that would govern how deep structure was transformed into the surface structure.

Syntax trees

Figure 3.4 illustrates a 'syntax tree' for sentence (4) – a simple, active sentence. Clearly, more complex sentences with subordinate and embedded

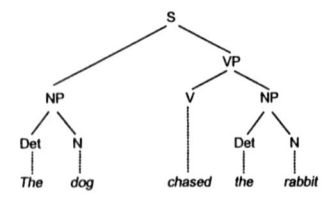

Fig. 3.4. An example of a 'syntax tree'

clauses will have correspondingly more complex syntax trees. Analyses of these have been used in the studies by Morice & Ingram (1982), subsequently replicated by a group in Edinburgh (e.g. Fraser *et al*, 1986). In these, speech transcripts were subjected to a computerised linguistic analysis after being converted into syntax trees. A variety of linguistic measures was thus derived, such as complexity of speech, mean number of embedded clauses per sentence, and semantic and syntactic errors. The original study compared schizophrenic, manic, and non-psychotic subjects, and using the measures patient groups could be distinguished with 95% accuracy using a discriminant function analysis. Subsequent studies have extended the approach, for instance, comparing subjects with negative symptoms with those with positive symptoms (Thomas *et al*, 1987). Overall, they illustrate well the potential contribution of formal linguistics in understanding disordered speech.

Semantics

The difference between semantics and syntax is immediately evident in the 'artificial' sentence:

(6) Colourless green ideas sleep furiously. (Chomsky, 1957)

Native speakers of English will recognise instantly that this is an odd construction. Equally, however, only a little further consideration will reveal that anomalous as it is, the sentence still seems to obey basic syntactic or grammatical rules – adjectives precede the noun, an adverb follows the verb, there is a recognisable subject–verb–object sequence. It is the *meaning* links between words that is disturbed. How can anything be colourless *and* green at the same time? Sleeping furiously sounds inherently contradictory. This is the field of semantics – the study of meaning in language.

'Meaning' itself has a number of meanings or connotations, however, in everyday use. If we ask "What is the meaning of life?", we are probably not asking for a definition of the last word in the sentence, but rather guidance on the point or purpose of existence. If we ask "What does the word *life* mean?", it is a definition we seek – what does this word refer to in the world? Semantics is concerned with this – how words in isolation or in sentence patterns carry meaning about the world.

Linguists have introduced the term 'lexeme' to represent the basic semantic unit. Why will 'word' not do for this? Firstly, take the examples *jumps, jumped, jumping, jumper*. These are clearly recognised as different words, yet there is a common underlying meaning unit, 'jump' – this would be the lexeme or lexical item. Secondly, there are many examples where a combination of several words may represent one underlying meaning unit, such as 'under the weather' for 'poorly', or 'kick the bucket' for 'die'. Here one lexeme contains three words.

Once again space precludes a full discussion of this interesting area, but a good introductory account can be found in the *Cambridge Encyclopaedia of Language* (Crystal, 1987).

Discourse and text

Much linguistic study has focused on understanding the construction of sentences. Increasingly, however, it is recognised that a full understanding of language function needs to take account of the way meaning is organised in the continuous sequence of sentences found in natural communication. A series of sentences should form a coherent whole, and in the Gestalt tradition, the whole discourse usually adds up to more than the sum of its parts.

'Discourse analysis' usually refers to the study of extended stretches of natural spoken language, whereas 'text analysis' is usually taken to refer to samples of written language. Confusingly, the terms are often used interchangeably, each referring to both written and spoken language (linguists do not appear phobic of ambiguous terminology!).

A particularly fruitful line of inquiry has been cohesion analysis, as described by Halliday & Hasan (1976). Essentially, this examines the interdependency of different sentences in a text by focusing on so-called 'cohesive ties'. These are the devices used to link the elements in different sentences that rely on one another for full comprehension. They are exemplified by 'anaphoric' references.

Take these two pairs of sentences:

(7) Have you seen my pencil?
(8) I've been looking for *it*.

(9) The computer failed and the telephone rang.
(10) *It* annoyed me.

In the first pair of sentences, the impersonal pronoun 'it' is used to stand for the object introduced in (7) – 'my pencil'. (Such devices appear to be used to avoid tedious repetition and improve the efficiency of communication.) The 'it' in (8) cannot be understood without referring to its correlate in (7). This is the anaphoric (backward-looking) relationship. The process can break down, however, as in the second pair of sentences. Here the impersonal pronoun could equally refer to either the computer or the telephone, leaving an ambiguity in the listener's or the reader's mind. Such errors rapidly lead to a text losing its coherence.

Rochester and colleagues (e.g. Rochester & Martin, 1979) have used this approach to examine schizophrenic language, and suggested that ambiguous referents are encountered more frequently in the speech of schizophrenics, particularly those manifesting clinical thought disorder. Furthermore, there appears to be difficulty in how schizophrenic speakers manipulate new and given information for the listener. For example, if in the course of a conversation I utter "Well, it's time to go now – where did I put that coat?", the use of "that coat" would lead the listener to suppose that the item in question has been mentioned earlier. Schizophrenic patients have a tendency to use such constructions when the information has *not* been given earlier.

These sorts of observations have led many investigators to suggest that a core feature of the disturbance in schizophrenic speech is a failure to take the listener's needs into account. That is, when planning or editing utterances, a schizophrenic person has difficulty taking the part of the listener and gauging whether the communication will be clear – which notably can be seen as a correlate of the clinical notion of autism.

In an interesting development from cohesion analysis, Wykes (1981) showed that clinical psychiatrists taught a basic approach to identifying cohesive ties were better able to distinguish transcripts of schizophrenic speech from that of manic patients. This is one of a few examples where linguistic techniques have been put directly to use in clinical practice, and it illustrates the potential applicability of psycholinguistic insights for the practitioner.

Pragmatics

This is the most recently developed level of linguistic inquiry, and it may be particularly pertinent to understanding the disturbance of communication in some patients. Returning to Fig. 3.1, pragmatics can be taken to represent the interface between the structural aspects of language and the actual *use* to which that structure is put – the factors that govern the practicalities of how language is actually used in social interaction.

Are not the structure and the use equivalent? An example where this is not the case is in so-called 'conversational implicature'. Imagine a junior doctor arriving breathless, ten minutes late for the ward round. The consultant asks "Do you know what time it is?" In this circumstance, the junior is most unlikely to assume the boss has forgotten to wear a watch and needs to know the time. More likely, the trainee will correctly assume the utterance to convey something like "Don't be late again if you want a career in psychiatry". This implicature is computed taking into account the circumstances, the relevant social standings, and prior knowledge of the speaker. This is one aspect of the pragmatics of language use.

H. P. Grice, who coined the term 'conversational implicature', has also been influential in describing some of the factors which appear to underlie successful verbal communication (e.g. Grice, 1975). He supposed that there was a general 'cooperative principle' shared by the participants in a communication: "any contribution to the conversational exchange is presumed to correspond to what is demanded of the speaker by the objective of this exchange" – that is, contributions should be goal-directed. In turn, Grice suggested that this cooperation rested on four basic 'conversational maxims' which, it is hoped, the participants will obey:

(a) the maxim of quality – say only what is true and what you know to be true
(b) the maxim of quantity – say no more and no less than is required
(c) the maxim of relation – be relevant
(d) the maxim of manner – be perspicuous (be brief and orderly; avoid obscurity and ambiguity).

For the most part, these maxims are unspoken. Sometimes they will not entirely be adhered to. For instance, the maxims may be deliberately flouted – as when we say "Lovely weather we're having . . ." on a cold, rainy day in June. Sarcastic effect is intended. At other times, the cooperation may *accidentally* break down. If spotted, this should lead to some attempt at so-called 'conversational repair' – the participants will cross-check or clarify, as in "I'm sorry, I forgot to mention that earlier". If not spotted, the participants may go on talking at cross-purposes.

Another aspect of pragmatics deals with how language is tailored to specific cultures and social situations. An example would be the distinction between the polite and familiar pronouns in French – *'vous'* and *'tu'*. Another is the ways in which language styles change between different circumstances of discourse. Consider your reaction if the following appeared in this chapter:

(11) The present author considers pragmatics to be central to understanding disordered communication

or

(12) I think pragmatics is important . . .

Many would think that the use of 'I' jars in scientific writing, the reader usually expecting to be distanced from the author in a serious piece by the (albeit stilted) use of something like "the present author".

In many other ways we modify our language style according to the social circumstances we are in: we speak very differently to patients, colleagues, children, or the supermarket checkout assistant.

Finally, mention could be made of the work done on 'speech acts'. J. L. Austin, a British philosopher, highlighted the fact that utterances can perform other functions than merely conveying information. In some situations an utterance can amount to an action – as in "I name this ship . . .". Expressing this actually changes the state of something, as does "You're fired," "I apologise for that," or "I guarantee you'll pass".

Speech acts may have an indirect quality reminiscent of conversational implicature. For instance, if we want someone to turn off the television, we might say "Turn off the television please," but, equally, any of these may get the same result: "I've seen this before," "Did we finish that game of Scrabble?" "There's a good concert on the radio". Even a loud yawn might suffice!

Pragmatics is a broad domain, then, with as yet ill-defined boundaries. Studies in the area overlap with discourse analysis, semantics, and sociolinguistics. Most would consider it be an overarching domain interacting with probably all the levels discussed in this chapter. It is likely that pragmatic elements will prove important in understanding at least some of the communication disturbance in mentally ill subjects, although as yet relatively few studies in the area have taken into account this level of analysis.

Acknowledgements

Thanks are due to Mrs Shirley Robinson, High Royds Hospital, for her invaluable secretarial assistance. The author is indebted to Cambridge University Press for permission to reproduce Fig. 3.2 from the *Cambridge Encyclopaedia of Language*.

References

CHAIKA, E. (1982) Thought disorder or speech disorder in schizophrenia? *Schizophrenia Bulletin*, **8**, 587–591.
CHOMSKY, A. N. (1957) *Syntactic Structures*. The Hague: Mouton.
CRYSTAL, D. (ed.) (1987) *The Cambridge Encyclopaedia of Language*. Cambridge: Cambridge University Press.
FRASER, W. I., KENDELL, R. E., KING, K., *et al* (1986) The diagnosis of schizophrenia by language analysis. *British Journal of Psychiatry*, **148**, 275–278.
FURTH, H. G. (1961) The influence of language on the development of concept formation in deaf children. *Journal of Abnormal and Social Psychology*, **63**, 386–389.

GRICE, H. P. (1975) Logic and conversation. In *Syntax and Semantics, Vol. 3, Speech Acts* (eds P. Cole & J. L. Morgan). New York: Seminar Press.
HALLIDAY, M. A. K. & HASAN, R. (1976) *Cohesion in English*. London: Longman.
MAHER, B. (1972) The language of schizophrenia: a review and interpretation. *British Journal of Psychiatry*, **120**, 3–17.
MALINOWSKI, B. (1972) Phatic communication. In *Communication in Face to Face Interaction* (eds J. Laver & S. Hutcheson), pp. 146–152. Baltimore: Penguin Books.
MORICE, R. D. & INGRAM, J. C. L. (1982) Language analysis in schizophrenia: diagnostic implications. *Australian and New Zealand Journal of Psychiatry*, **16**, 11–21.
ROCHESTER, S. R. & MARTIN, J. R. (1979) *Crazy Talk: A Study of the Discourse of Schizophrenic Speakers*. New York: Plenum Press.
SLOBIN, D. I. (1979) *Psycholinguistics* (2nd edn). Glenview, Ill.: Scott Foresman.
THOMAS, P., KING, K. & FRASER, W. I. (1987) Postive and negative symptoms of schizophrenia and linguistic performance. *Acta Psychiatrica Scandinavica*, **76**, 144–151.
WEBSTER'S THIRD NEW INTERNATIONAL DICTIONARY (1961) New York: Merriam-Webster.
WYKES, T. (1981) Can the psychiatrist learn from the psychologist? Detecting coherence in the disordered speech of manics and schizophrenics. *Psychological Medicine*, **11**, 641–642.

Part II. Schizophrenic disturbance of speech and language

4 On analysing schizophrenic speech: what model should we use?

ELAINE CHAIKA

Why do we judge the unusual oral creations of some schizophrenic people as being speech disordered? It cannot be simply because they are unusual or because they are new creations. After all, language is nothing if it is not creative. Any speaker can make up new words, use old words in new ways, play with the sounds and syntax of the language, make words shift from one part of speech to another, and still be considered perfectly normal, or even a genius. Nobody is bound by some abstract set of rules which generate only the sentences of his or her language, nor by inviolable rules for word usage. If we were, then the words and syntax of language would not change as rapidly as they do. That is why we do not speak the language of Fielding or even of Dickens, and it is why we Americans have managed to make our varieties of English so divergent from the British in a mere three centuries. The essence of language is that it is not static. Differentness cannot explain why we consider some schizophrenic verbal productions disordered or incompetent.

Linguists are learning that language responds to cognitive and pragmatic forces, and these provide better models for verbal productions than do models depending on the syntactic generation of sentences (Hoffman & Sledge, 1984). The very development of syntactic categories in all languages is as strongly influenced by pragmatic forces as it is by syntactic rules. Heine *et al* (1991) have found this to be as true in African languages, as Ruwet (1991) has found it to be true in French and English. Even such fundamentals of language as the parts of speech can be shown to be changeable by pragmatic strategies. Heine *et al* found that in African languages prepositions could become nouns or verbs under the right circumstances. We see this in English, as when we say "Up the ante," changing the preposition to a verb, or "It has its ups and downs," treating the prepositions as nouns. Linguists have long been aware that there are fuzzy borders for all syntactic categories and for all rules of language.

Human language is not *isomorphic*. That is, there is no one-to-one equivalence between message and meaning. Much, if not most, meaning is effected by metaphor, which we now know is a matter of control of visual as well as of semantic processes. We can metaphorically indicate a meaning with words and phrases far different from what they say, so long as they conform to our visual images, or our cognitive models (Lakoff & Johnson, 1980; Lakoff, 1987), both cultural and individual. Lakoff & Johnson have shown, for instance, that even such strange imagery as "My mother will have a cow" or "Jack flipped his lid" works because of our knowledge of what it feels like to be angry and that, so long as metaphors for anger conform to images of building up pressure, something inside the body bursting to come out, visual impairment, becoming red-faced, and other physical correlates of anger, we can produce new metaphors for anger. These may on the surface seem bizarre, but are not taken as bizarre by speakers of English, for instance. That is, we unthinkingly process what are actually outlandish images – that of a person giving birth to a cow or of the top of someone's head blowing off – as if they are as straightforward as saying "Roses are red". It is such interplay between cognition, strategy, and cultural conventions which makes language so infinitely creative.

It is when we hear verbal productions by fellow speakers of our language(s) as bizarre or confused that we know we are facing true speech disorder. For this population, it appears as if the creative processes built into speakers have gone awry.

In the face of what we know about pragmatic and cognitive constraints on language and its production, some linguists, including me, no longer believe that there is an abstract pure *langue* as opposed to *parole*. Increasingly, my studies into language, deviant and normal, over the past quarter century, have led me to believe that language is speech. Language is being created anew by individual speakers all the time. Syntax, along with every other facet of language, is constantly in a state of becoming something else. Daily, numberless nonce forms are being produced and heard as normal language. Still, nonce forms in speech disorder strike listeners as being deviant, as caused by a psychopathology. The question is, what is the nature of this pathology?

When I first approached this problem, it seemed to me that schizophrenic speech might be aphasic. There certainly are parallels in verbal production between those two populations. However, undeniably, there are times when speech-disordered schizophrenic subjects speak normally, or at least so that nobody finds their productions deviantly structured, and some schizophrenic people seem not to produce aphasia-like output at all. Furthermore, they do not necessarily show true aphasic dysfunction in aphasic battery tests. In short, there is no real proof that there is any disruption in basic language competence in schizophrenia, although there may be other generalised cognitive or performance disabilities. At the same time, the constellation of errors associated with specifically schizophrenic speech are not likely to be under voluntary control (Chaika, 1982, 1990; Chaika & Alexander, 1986).

Output and intention

One need not go far in the literature before encountering genuine disruptions in syntactic production in schizophrenia, but one also finds recognisably schizophrenic output which is syntactically skilful, such as Maher's (1983) famous example:

> "If you think you are being wise to send me a bill for money I have already paid I am in nowise going to do so unless I get the whys and wherefores from you to me. But where fours have been, then fives will be, and other numbers and calculations and accounts to your no-account no-bill, noble, nothing."

Such examples may lead one to conclude that schizophrenic people have diminished competence in performance or in effecting creativity. However, the syntax of this passage is not only normal, but evinces several complex structures correctly executed.[1]

Nor can such speech be explained by such concepts as 'loosening of constructs' or unusual word associations, two common explanations in the past. No construct in language is hard and fast. Every word, indeed, every construction, is inherently elastic, and it is the *fact* of associating that makes schizophrenic speech peculiar. Normal speech is never produced on the basis of word associations. If there is one trait that is pathognomic of speech disorder in schizophrenia and mania, it is the chaining of phrases on the basis of semantic or phonological associations, as in the following identification of a colour chip:

> "Looks like clay. Sounds like grey. Take you for a roll in the hay. Hay day. May day. Help. I need help." (Cohen, 1978)

Such speech seems to suffer from path control. That is, schizophrenic people typically start out most of their utterances somewhere at least near where one would assume a target should be, but then veer off on associated pathways (Chaika, 1982). This apparently remains true regardless of how speech data are collected, whether from free speech or speech produced under various test conditions. One hypothesis which accounts for such speech is that there is a lapse between intention and output, combined with a deficit in self-monitoring, at least at the time that the disordered speech was produced. The intention is shown by the first part of the utterance.

In order to investigate intention, one must give speakers a target towards which they should be aiming. Provided there is evidence that schizophrenic subjects are cooperating in the experimental task, then their output can be

---

1. The first sentence alone contains a conditional clause, a verbal complement clause, a relative clause, a main clause, and another conditional. See Chaika (1990, pp. 229–230) for further discussion of this passage and the specific dysfunction it represents.

matched with that of normals to see the nature of the mismatch between intention and output. Rochester & Martin (1979) did just that, eliciting narratives under free and controlled situations. Considering that schizophrenic speech is quite disjointed, they hypothesised that this population did not use cohesive ties properly. Consequently, their guide for analysis was Halliday & Hasan's (1976) exhaustive treatment of the devices we use in English to make sentences cohere with each other to form discourses. This certainly is a reasonable approach, and one which had to be attempted.

An empirical study

For the most part, Rochester & Martin found that schizophrenic subjects did not greatly differ from normal subjects in their use of cohesive ties, although they were more likely to use exophora (reference to something in the environment) rather than anaphora (reference back to something just said). However, this finding, although interesting, is not really explanatory, because neither device, anaphora or exophora, leads to coherence or incoherence. It is how these devices are used, not their number, which determines coherence. A passage can be loaded with cohesive ties and still be incoherent. For instance, in the following fragment from a schizophrenic narrator (Chaika & Alexander, 1986; Chaika, 1990), note the number of cohesive ties (in boldface):

"... **Her** parents **that she**'s so proud of **she** goes out, leaves the ice cream **and** eats **it and** on the way **and** we don't know what happens the fact. You can interpolate and say **that she** ate the ice cream **and** brought it home...."

Throughout this narrative, the patient correctly uses all pronouns, like *she* and *her*. Additionally, he uses *the* correctly to indicate nouns previously mentioned. Still, the narrative is not coherent.

These data were collected in a study of normal, schizophrenic, and manic narration in a tightly bound situation. All diagnoses of schizophrenia and mania were based upon DSM–II and DSM–III by the attending physicians at Butler Hospital, Brown University. Subjects, matched for age, occupation, education, and social class, individually viewed a 124-second video story entitled "The Ice Cream Story" (Chaika & Alexander, 1986; Chaika, 1990). Then each was directed to tell the investigator what he or she had just seen. (The video story has been extensively described elsewhere.)

Every subject showed intention to retell the story which they had just viewed. For instance, all included events of the video story in their narratives, and even highly deviant schizophrenic narratives concluded with expressions of satisfaction that the speaker believed he or she had told the story. It was thus possible to distinguish intention from production. These results suggested a failure of self-monitoring.

This narrative task (Chaika, 1990, pp. 133–145) uncovered no significant difference in number of errors overall of any sort between normal and schizophrenic subjects, nor did it reveal a statistically significant difference in the number of cohesive ties which each population used. Even the kinds of cohesive ties used by each population were not significantly different. There were no significant differences between the populations in the numbers and types of dysfluencies: stuttering, hesitating, starting a sentence and breaking it off. Nor was there a difference between them in the number of misperceptions they recorded in the task. Surprisingly, normal subjects were not significantly more accurate than schizophrenic and manic subjects in retelling the story.

What were different, however, were the kinds of errors, dysfluencies and misperceptions each population had. These showed differential patterns for normal subjects, on the one hand, and schizophrenic and manic subjects, on the other, with, in every instance, schizophrenic subjects differing from manic and normal subjects in severity of dysfunction.

Specifically, when normal subjects misperceived, the misperception still fitted into a story line, but schizophrenic misperceptions had no relation to the rest of the story. For instance, several normal subjects said the icecream was chocolate, when it was grape ice. This did not change the main point of the story in any way, however: the flavour of the ice-cream was immaterial. However, a schizophrenic subject said that the girl was moving a display case in the shop, when, in fact, she was simply leaning up against it. Both normal and psychotic subjects digressed, and did so a similar number of times. However, whenever the normal subjects digressed, they indicated that they were doing so, and went back to the main narrative:

> "and then she [intonation remains at high level; pause] – her father came home from work, **whatever** – [pause] she asked her father for money." (Chaika, 1990, p. 199)

In contrast, psychotic subjects just veered off the story line and often never went back to it (Chaika, 1990, p. 206), creating the narrative equivalent of glossomanic chaining. Similarly, schizophrenic, but not normal subjects, would begin a constituent structure and simply not finish it, as in:

> "He was blamed **for** and I don't think that was fair the way they did that either.
> What are **the** and uh there was a scene.
> Another car **pulls** and then a little girl is peeking."

It must be emphasised that errors like these were not exclusive to psychotic subjects, but they were said as if nothing had been omitted. There was no break in intonation and stress. The word vital to a syntactic construction was simply omitted.

Normal subjects, in contrast, would break off in the middle of a syntactic construction, but they signalled that they were going to do so or had done so. Moreover, in every case, they produced a completed construction which fit into the narrative:

> "... and it wasn't really ice cream she wanted, it was – **uh she ordered frozen grape ice, a double order.**" (Chaika, 1990, p. 205)

Slips of the tongue

One might be tempted to argue that the fact of not completing constituent structures is a deficit in syntax; however, even those psychotic subjects who evince such error often *did* complete their constituent structures correctly. There is another explanation for non-completion, one which accords with the constellation of errors made by schizophrenic people (Chaika, 1982). For this, we should look at the intensive research into slip-of-the-tongue phenomena. Baars (1992) concludes that such slips are caused by a lapse between volition and performance, and are ultimately caused by a temporary malfunction of the executive function of the brain. Werner *et al*'s (1975) suggestion that schizophrenic people do not self-monitor correctly, also put forth by Chaika (1990, p. 58) and Frith (1992), is consistent with this account of slips of the tongue. Scholars like Fodor (1983) and Gazzaniga (1992) hypothesise that the mind is modular. In turn, this entails the existence of an executive function (or interpreter) which selects and coordinates the modules. In particular, Gazzaniga's results with 'split-brain' patients are difficult to explain without such a presumption. Volition must exist apart from this executive function, as it determines what the executive will be selecting.

A great deal of support for such a theory comes from research into slips of the tongue. MacKay (1992) points out that most of the nodes in our minds are full of unconscious knowledge and skills. An executive decides what will get put into the consciousness. He points out that creativity requires formation of new connections between nodes. Often when these are activated, some processes remain unconscious. An example is the unconscious selection of the correct pronunciation of the plural of a word, even when the word's meaning itself may be conscious. For instance, if one says "track cowz" when one meant "cow tracks" the executive has chosen the right words for the intended production, but something has gone wrong with production itself so that the words have been transposed. When this happens, the plural goes on 'cow' rather than 'track', but the speaker uses the [z] sound which is appropriate for the plural of 'cow' rather than the [s] which is appropriate for the intended plural of 'track'. This is an unconscious choice. When the time comes to put on the plural, one's internal monitor allows it to be put on the actually uttered word, even though the speaker did not intend to pluralise that word. Invariably, when this happens, the right ending is attached, albeit on the wrong word. The speaker may be aware of the slip of the tongue, but not the particular variant of the plural actually used. There is a good deal of evidence of such lack of awareness in slips of the tongue, evidence of automated rules operating even when the words chosen are not the ones intended. That is, the wrong word(s) get the right rules.

It must be noted that automated phonological rules such as these are essentially syntactic rules. Schizophrenic subjects, like normal subjects, typically apply such rules correctly even when creating nonsense words or gibberish (Chaika, 1977). If MacKay is correct, and there is no reason to doubt his observations, then we can understand schizophrenic error in terms of slips of the tongue. For instance, not only do schizophrenic subjects use automated phonological rules correctly on the wrong words, but schizophrenic errors are often contained in correct syntactic frames, such as in the segment quoted above, "Looks like clay. Sounds like grey." Here, the wrong word 'grey', is in the same kind of syntactic frame as the appropriate 'looks like', which refers to visual phenomena. Moreover, this opening statement was correct. The colour chip the patient was identifying was clay coloured. 'Sounds like' is the same sort of syntactic construction, and belongs in the same set of verbs referring to the senses as does 'looks like', but it does not fit the context. It appears there has been an automatic generation of related syntactic constructions into which a word related to the target word, 'clay', has been inserted (Chaika, 1982). Such automatic generation of syntactic rules explains why we do not usually get just strings of related words in glossomania. Glossomanic chains typically are related words ensconced in syntactic frames.

Garrett (1980) shows that when the executive is looking for a word with a given meaning in line with intention, it may access all the meanings of the words chosen, even ones inappropriate to the context, or it may access many words with the same meaning rather than one. This is a picture of what occurs in schizophrenic glossomania. The pathology lies in the degree to which the subject is unable to ignore the superfluous words and to suppress their production.

Reason (1984) claims that whenever words depart from their planned course, they tend to do so in the direction of producing something more familiar, and in keeping with existing knowledge structures and immediate surroundings, rather than that which was originally intended. This, simply stated, is a succinct summary of schizophrenic narrative wandering.

Baars and others have found that slips of the tongue cannot be explained by errors in applying transformational or other linguistic rules. There is a limited amount of space for consciousness, which sits upon a much larger amount of unconscious knowledge and skills. It has been shown in a wide variety of laboratory experiments that if the consciousness is presented with competing plans, these plans cause slips of the tongue and even slips in action. These are either a combination of the competing plans or an activation of automatic processes which are inappropriate for the matter at hand.

Baars claims that errors may also be caused by lapses in consciousness, and gives convincing evidence that such errors are involuntary. This body of research, which is far more extensive than I can report here, encompasses both naturally occurring slips and those induced in the laboratory. Either source yields data which, in many respects, but not all, are remarkably like disordered speech. Normal subjects produce unintended puns, neologisms, and words related phonologically or semantically to target words, such as 'play' for 'stay', 'homofering interphones' for 'interfering homophones', or 'horricle mirable' for 'horrible miracle'. Error in speech disorder is not necessarily so transparent or so close to the mark as normal error (Chaika, 1977), although the result is inappropriate rhyming, "That's all I can *stew*", non-words composed of recognisable morphemes, "*puterience, duocratic*", and outright neologising, "He had *fooch* with *tey kraimz* I'll be willin' to betcha". Additionally, in the ice-cream stories noted above, although both normal and schizophrenic subjects stuttered on the initial sound of a word occasionally, only schizophrenic stuttering was followed by a word with a different phoneme from the eventual word uttered, as in "He ch-told", whereas normal subjects produced "f-f-for" (Chaika, 1990, pp. 199–200).

As has long been noted (Fromkin, 1971), using an antonym of a target word, or the wrong word of a set, such as 'stove' for 'refrigerator', are common slips of the tongue. These have their counterparts in schizophrenic "opposite speech", which can be seen as a more severe form of lapse in antonym selection (Laffal, 1965; Chaika, 1977). Since both the normal and schizophrenic error do show some relation to the target, we can assume the same cause of error in each population, although schizophrenic error is less controlled than normal, and veers more chaotically from the target.

At least one kind of schizophrenic error does not seem to occur in normal subjects, even when errors are deliberately induced in the laboratory. MacKay (1992, p. 53) notes that normal subjects never make 'garden path' errors, or what we term the glossomanic chains in schizophrenic speech disorder. However, glossomania is not necessarily different in kind from normal error. It is as reasonable to assume that they are different only in degree. Glossomanic chains seem to be especially persistent errors in accessing target words and in suppressing related words which are activated along with targets. This conforms to the fact that schizophrenic error is generally more disorganised and more persistent than normal slips.

Conclusions

Given the intermittent nature of speech disorder, rather than considering it as a kind of aphasia, it is more fruitful to consider it as a lapse in volition, as Baars and others say normal slips are. That is, we can posit the same causation for speech disorder as for normal slips, except that the errors in speech disorder are more persistent and more disorganised. The difference seems to be that the executive controller, which selects items for output on the basis of volition, has more severe lapses in consciousness in schizophrenia.

This conclusion is a departure from my original assumptions about the aetiology of schizophrenic speech, assumptions then based upon a Chomskyan perception of language, one that investigation no longer supports. I no longer think that error in speech disorder should be necessarily equated with the aphasias which result from actual brain damage. (This does not necessarily mean that schizophrenic speech disorder is not a kind of aphasia; it is just that the facts support the conclusion that it is caused by a lapse in volition and executive control.)

Nor do I see speech disorder, or even normal slips, as being necessarily caused by misapplication of linguistic rules. To claim this is to beg the question of why people misapply rules, rules which they are not conscious of applying in the first place.[2]

Determining the appropriate way to analyse speech disorder is not a trivial matter. The interpretation of meaning of such speech can be quite different according to whether it is perceived as resulting from a true deficit in language production as opposed to resulting from failed intention. The degree to which the actual verbal output will even be heeded can depend upon diagnosis. The research on slips has gone a long way in uncovering the disparity between target and production, showing the directions in which errors occur. Therefore, if the slip-of-the-tongue model for schizophrenia is viable, then this research promises to give us firmer foundation for interpreting speech disorder.

References

BAARS, B. (ed.) (1992) *Experimental Slips and Human Error: Exploring the Architecture of Volition.* New York: Plenum Press.

---

2. Normals do not recognise up to 40% of the slips they make, although if these are pointed out, they can then recognise their errors, and even repeat the errors, whereas schizophrenic subjects seem not to be able to recognise their errors, much less to repeat them when they are pointed out. However, some schizophrenic subjects do comment on the fact that they are aware of having generalised difficulty in talking. In the ice-cream stories study (Chaika, 1990), I allowed all subjects to play back the tape recordings of their narratives, but schizophrenic and manic subjects never made any sign that they noticed their dysfluencies, no matter how jarring.

CHAIKA, E. (1977) Schizophrenic speech, slips of the tongue, and jargonaphasia: a reply to Fromkin and to Lecours and Vaniers-Clement. *Brain and Language*, **4**, 464–475.
—— (1982) A unified explanation for the diverse structural deviations reported for adult schizophrenics with disrupted speech. *Journal of Communication Disorders*, **15**, 167–189.
—— (1990) *Understanding Psychotic Speech: Beyond Freud and Chomsky*. Springfield: Charles C. Thomas.
—— & ALEXANDER, P. (1986) The ice cream stories: a study in normal and psychotic narrations. *Discourse Processes*, **9**, 305–328.
COHEN, B. (1978) Referent communication disturbances in schizophrenia. In *Language and Cognition in Schizophrenia* (ed. S. Schwartz), pp. 1–34. Hillsdale: Lawrence Erlbaum.
FODER, J. (1983) *The Modularity of Mind: An Essay into Faculty Psychology*. Cambridge: MIT Press.
FRITH, C. (1992) *The Cognitive Neuropsychology of Schizophrenia*. Hillsdale: Lawrence Erlbaum.
FROMKIN, V. (1971) The non-anomalous nature of anomalous utterances. *Language*, **47**, 27–52.
GARRETT, M. F. (1980) The limits of accommodation: arguments for independent processing levels in sentence production. In *Errors in Linguistic Performance: Slips of the Tongue, Ear, Pen, and Hand* (ed. V. Fromkin), pp. 263–271. New York: Academic Press.
GAZZANIGA, M. (1992) *Nature's Mind: The Biological Roots of Thinking, Emotions, Sexuality, Language, and Intelligence*. New York: Basic Books.
HALLIDAY, M. & HASAN, R. (1976) *Cohesion in English*. London: Longman.
HEINE, B., CLAUDI, U. & HUNNEMEYER, F. (1991) *Grammaticalization: A Conceptual Framework*. Chicago: University of Chicago Press.
HOFFMAN, R. & SLEDGE, W. (1984) A microgenetic model of paragrammatisms produced by a schizophrenic speaker. *Brain and Language*, **21**, 147–173.
LAFFAL, J. (1965) *Pathological and Normal Language*. New York: Atherton Press.
LAKOFF, G. (1987) *Women, Fire and Dangerous Things: What Categories Reveal about the Mind*. Chicago: University of Chicago Press.
—— & JOHNSON, M. (1980) *Metaphors We Live By*. Chicago: University of Chicago Press.
MACKAY, D. (1992) Errors, ambiguity, and awareness in language perception and production. In *Experimental Slips and Human Error: Exploring the Architecture of Volition* (ed. B. Baars), pp. 438–506. New York: Plenum Press.
MAHER, B. (1983) A tentative theory of schizophrenic utterance. *Progress in Experimental Personality Research*, Vol. 12. New York: Academic Press.
REASON, J. (1984). Lapses of attention in everyday life. In *Varieties of Attention* (eds R. Parasuraman & D. R. Davies), pp. 515–549. New York: Academic Press.
ROCHESTER, S. & MARTIN, J. (1979) *Crazy Talk: A Study of the Discourse of Schizophrenic Speakers*. New York: Plenum Press.
RUWET, N. (1991) *Syntax and Human Experience* (ed. and trans. J. Goldsmith). Chicago: University of Chicago Press.
WERNER, O., LEWIS-MATICHEK, G., EVANS, M., *et al* (1975) An ethnoscience view of schizophrenic speech. In *Sociocultural Dimensions of Language Use* (eds M. Sanches & B. Blount), pp. 349–380. Oakland: Scott, Foresman.

5 Language impairments and executive dysfunction in schizophrenia

RODNEY MORICE

It is not controversial to make a claim for speech and language impairments in schizophrenia. They have been described frequently, using a variety of constructs, since the seminal descriptions of Kraepelin (1919) and Bleuler (1950). Somewhat more controversial have been the imputed relationships between speech and language impairments and thought, in particular thought disorder. These relationships are not the topic of this chapter. Interpretations of the speech and language impairments have also engendered controversy, and these are the topic. As the final interpretation offered will be largely speculative, further controversy is likely to accrue.

Early interpretations

Kraepelin and Bleuler differed fundamentally in their interpretations of the speech and language impairments they described. Kraepelin adopted a more anatomical perspective, possibly influenced by the writings of Broca (1863) and Wernicke (1874) in relation to neurological impairments of speech and language. He clearly described telegrammatic speech as well as paraphasias and neologisms, the former similar to agrammatic, or Broca's, aphasia, and the latter to fluent, or Wernicke's aphasia.

While Bleuler acknowledged "every imaginable abnormality" in the "form of linguistic expression" (Bleuler, 1950, p. 148), he did not place importance on the speech changes as such, giving primacy to thought, or conceptual, confusion. Accordingly, he did not seek to localise speech impairments, but rather to provide a functional interpretation. A disturbance in the associations between thoughts comprised the first of his *fundamental* symptoms (symptoms characteristic of schizophrenia), as well as one of the *primary* symptoms ("stemming directly from the disease process itself", p. 348), while disorders of speech comprised only the fifth of his *accessory* symptoms (symptoms also occurring in other disorders).

Kraepelin's interpretations were supported by Kleist (1960). He described two distinct patterns of syntactic change, one an agrammatic form characterised by omitted function words and simple sentences, and the other a paragrammatic form characterised paraphasias, neologisms, and long, complex, often unfinished sentences. The former pattern Kleist attributed to a type of anterior, or motor, aphasia, and the latter to a posterior, or sensory, aphasia. This dichotomy, based on the presumed primary language centres in the brain, influenced many subsequent interpretations and debate as to whether language impairment in schizophrenia reflected one, the other, or both, types of aphasia.

Both approaches, Kraepelinian/Kleistian and Bleulerian, to the interpretation of speech and language impairments in schizophrenia have influenced, and perhaps constrained, research. The Bleulerian view, that thought disorder (in a broad sense) led to speech impairment, could have influenced the growth of psychodynamic and of semantic interpretations of speech impairment, arguably at the expense of detailed linguistic analyses and neuroanatomical hypothesis. The Kraepelinian view, especially with Kleist's subsequent developments, supported a dichotomous perspective of two distinct subtypes of speech and language impairment, preceding by decades Crow's (1980) type I and type II schizophrenias. This chapter attempts to draw these dichotomous approaches together.

Linguistic performance in schizophrenia

Without wishing to underestimate the clinical and possible theoretical importance of disorders of speech and thought content, my own earlier research concentrated on the syntax, or grammar, of schizophrenic speech. I set out initially to disprove the several then more recent assertions in the literature that there were no impairments of syntax in the speech of schizophrenic people (Rochester *et al*, 1973; Carpenter, 1976; Andreasen, 1982), the original descriptions of Kraepelin (1919), and even of Bleuler (1950), notwithstanding.

A computer-assisted analysis of manually parsed samples of free speech of 1000 words from each subject was used. Manual parsing produced syntax tree diagrams (Fig. 5.1) for each analysable sentence, with each tree containing, at the base, the identified parts of speech. Different levels of the syntax tree reflected levels of clausal embedding. During the manual parse, errors and dysfluencies also were tagged.

All information, including the actual tree diagrams, was entered into first an Apple, and later a NorthStar microcomputer. A suite of programs entitled PSYCHLAN produced a summary table of 118 linguistic variables for each subject. Most of these were not used in subsequent statistical analyses because of their infrequent occurrence in the samples.

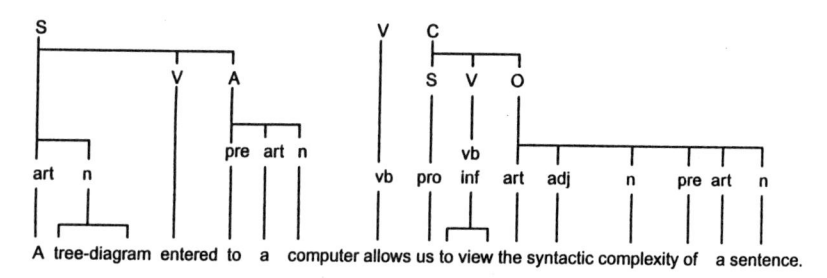

```
S                          V   C
├────┬─────┐               │   ├─────┬──────────────────┐
│    V     A               │   S  V  O
│    │   ┌─┴──┐            │   │  │  ├────┬────┬────┬────┬───┐
│    │   pre art n         │   │  vb │    │    │    │    │   │
art  n   │   │  │          vb  pro inf art adj  n   pre art  n
│    │   │   │  │          │   │  │  │    │    │    │    │   │
A tree-diagram entered to a computer allows us to view the syntactic complexity of a sentence.
```

Fig. 5.1. A syntax tree diagram: S, subject; V, verb; C, complement; A, adverbial clause; O, object; pre, preposition; art, article; n, noun; vb, verb; pro, pronoun; vb inf, infinitive verb; adj, adjective

Three separate studies now using this method of speech and language analysis have been able to discriminate between schizophrenic, manic and control subjects using selected linguistic variables, and with respectable diagnostic confidence (Morice & Ingram, 1982; Morice & McNicol, 1986; Fraser *et al*, 1986). In summary, the three studies, one in Adelaide, South Australia, one in Hobart, Tasmania, and an independent one in Edinburgh, Scotland, showed that schizophrenic subjects, as a group, uttered speech of reduced syntactic complexity, made more syntactic and semantic errors, and were more dysfluent than non-psychiatric control subjects. Manic subjects, as a group, tended to record linguistic profiles somewhere between those of the schizophrenic and control subjects.

While none of these studies, nor any of the subsequent studies by members of the original Edinburgh group (Thomas *et al*, 1987, 1990; King *et al*, 1990), reported correlations between the major linguistic variables, there did seem to be a 'trade-off' between the complexity of expressed speech and the number of errors. In other words, those speakers expressing syntactically simple sentences made few errors. As the complexity increased, so too did the number of errors. Some schizophrenic speakers produced extremely long sentences, but not infrequently they contained multiple errors, and many were unfinished. As one of the schizophrenic subjects in the first study expressed it, "and communicating ordinarily I can get lost in the chaos of the language" (Morice, 1986*a*).

This apparent 'trade-off' has been supported by a subsequent correlation analysis of relevant results from the two Australian studies. Thirty-three schizophrenic subjects, diagnosed according to Research Diagnostic Criteria for the 15 Adelaide subjects, and to DSM–III criteria for the 18 Hobart subjects, were contrasted with 37 non-psychiatric controls from both centres. Using a procedure similar to the Edinburgh group's (King *et al*, 1990), raw scores of selected variables were Z-transformed, and mean summated Z scores were used to produce composite syntactic complexity, syntactic/semantic integrity, and dysfluency scores.

The syntactic complexity score comprised Z scores for the following variables: mean length of utterance of analysable sentences, percentage of sentences with embedded clauses, mean number of embedded clauses per sentence, and mean depth of clausal embedding per sentence. The syntactic/semantic integrity (or error) score comprised: percentage of syntactically deviant sentences, percentage of semantically deviant sentences, number of word-level errors, and total number of errors. The dysfluency score comprised: percentage of pause fillers, percentage of false starts retraced, and percentage of repeat words and multiple-word repeats. Each composite variable was thought to reflect more comprehensively than any single variable could, the constructs of syntactic complexity, integrity, and dysfluency.

The correlation matrix (Pearson's r) for each group is displayed in Table 5.1. Separate group matrices were generated, as it was hypothesised that a 'trade-off' between complexity and integrity would be more marked for the schizophrenic group. There was a moderate, but significant, positive correlation between the complexity and integrity scores for the schizophrenic subjects only. In other words, for schizophrenic subjects, and not for controls, as the syntactic complexity of sentences increased, so did the number of errors. There was a shared variance of 23% between complexity and integrity, offering support for the 'trade-off' hypothesis. There were no significant correlations with dysfluency for either group.

Naturally, significant positive correlations could result if there were two clusters of speakers, the one producing syntactically simple sentences with few errors, and the other producing syntactically complex sentences containing many errors. Such clusters, if they existed, could be taken to support the dichotomy of language impairments into anterior and posterior subtypes.

However, examination of the stem-and-leaf plots for the complexity and integrity composite measures, and for each of the component variables, did not reveal bimodal distributions, such as would occur if there were two dichotomous groups. There were no distinct 'points of rarity' in the distributions of any of the variables.

TABLE 5.1
Correlation coefficients (Pearson's r) between composite linguistic variables

	Complexity	Integrity	Dysfluency
Schizophrenic group (n = 33)			
Complexity	1.00		
Integrity	0.48*	1.00	
Dysfluency	0.17	0.10	1.00
Control group (n = 37)			
Complexity	1.00		
Integrity	0.19	1.00	
Dysfluency	0.04	0.08	1.00

*$P < 0.01$, one-tailed significance.

Syntactic complexity and integrity measures appeared to comprise continuous, not dichotomous, variables, suggesting that language impairments in schizophrenia may not reflect variants of anterior and posterior aphasia, although the extremes at the end of each continuum, looked at separately, could naturally suggest two distinct subtypes.

The absence of dichotomous groups was also supported by an examination of the scatterplot of composite complexity and error scores for the schizophrenic and control subjects (Fig. 5.2). While control subjects were largely error free, and scattered along the complexity axis, schizophrenic subjects were distributed across three of the four quadrants. They did not group into two dichotomous clusters, nor were the three groupings widely separated from each other to suggest 'points of rarity'.

The suggestion of a 'trade-off' between complexity and integrity in speech and language motivated the creation of a 'linguistic performance' metric, to borrow Chomsky's (1965) term. While Chomsky's other familiar term, 'linguistic competence', referred to a speaker's innate knowledge of language, 'linguistic performance' referred to the actual production of speech, constrained as it might be by non-linguistic factors such as attention and memory, or indeed by working memory (Baddeley, 1986).

One of the essential features of competent linguistic performance must be the production of sentences of appropriate syntactic complexity, complex enough to transmit relevant information, while free from errors. The linguistic performance metric was computed for each subject by subtracting the composite integrity (error) score from the composite syntactic complexity score. The metric thus indicated the average transformed level of syntactic complexity for each subject that could be attained without error.

The validity of this metric was supported by the presence of significant correlations with the composite complexity and integrity variables, at 0.75 and −0.48 respectively. Additionally, the new metric correlated with greater

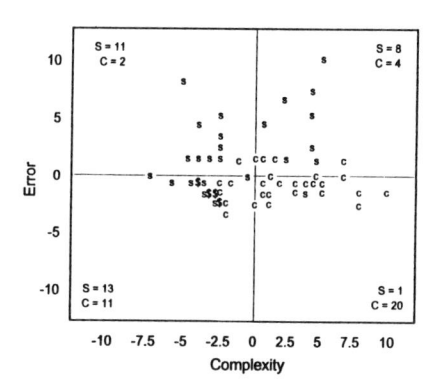

Fig. 5.2. *Language complexity and error distribution for schizophrenic (s) and control (c) subjects. ($) indicates multiple subjects*

TABLE 5.2
Correlation coefficients (Pearson's r) for transformed composite linguistic variables with scores on the token test for schizophrenic and control groups combined (n = 37)

	Complexity	Integrity	Linguistic performance	Part 7 of the token test	Token test total score
Complexity	1.00				
Integrity	0.21	1.00			
Linguistic performance	0.75**	−0.48*	1.00		
Part 7 of the token test	0.44*	−0.31	0.60**	1.00	
Token test total score	0.42*	−0.31	0.58**	0.98**	1.00

*$P<0.01$, **$P<0.001$, one-tailed significance.

strength than either of the composite variables with measures derived from the token test, a test for the comprehension of syntax (described below) (Table 5.2).

For both the schizophrenic and control groups, scores for linguistic performance were distributed normally, with little skew, and with no suggestion of points of rarity. Normality was confirmed by the Shapiro–Wilks statistic (0.96, d.f. = 37, $P = 0.39$), and unimodality by inspection of the stem-and-leaf plots.

Analysis of variance revealed a strongly significant difference between the scores for the two groups (Table 5.3). The schizophrenic subjects, as a group, were able only to produce relatively non-complex speech that was error free. Such speech, overall, might be expected to comprise a functional 'poverty of content of speech', in that because of the degree of syntactic simplicity, the content would be relatively bereft of meaning.

The linguistic performance of schizophrenic subjects, then, was significantly impaired, but within the group, the distribution of the metric was normal and unimodal. The composite measure of speech and language impairment did not suggest linguistic subtypes within the schizophrenic group.

Executive impairment in schizophrenia

If the language impairments in schizophrenia do not represent variants of Broca's and Wernicke's aphasias, how can they be explained? I suggest that they could be explained by a dysexecutive syndrome (Baddeley, 1986),

TABLE 5.3
Group means and analysis of variance results for scores for linguistic performance

	Mean (s.d.) score for linguistic performance	Analysis of variance
Schizophrenic subjects ($n = 33$)	−0.76 (0.93)	$F = 47.53$, d.f. = 1, 68, $P = 0.0000$
Control subjects ($n = 37$)	0.68 (0.81)	

impairments affecting executive functions arguably subserved by the prefrontal cortex and its distributed neural networks.

With my colleague, neuropsychologist Ann Delahunty, I have completed a study of executive impairments in schizophrenia. This followed a study (Morice, 1990) in which substantial impairments in cognitive flexibility were found in both schizophrenic and manic subjects. In the most recent study, we measured cognitive flexibility (using the Wisconsin card sorting test; Berg, 1948; Heaton, 1981), forward planning (using Tower of London; Shallice, 1982), and working memory (using sentence span; Daneman & Carpenter, 1980). Major impairments in all areas of functioning were demonstrated in the schizophrenic group ($n = 19$), as compared with non-psychiatric controls ($n = 19$). All schizophrenic subjects were living in the community at the time of testing, with 16 (84.2%) stabilised on antipsychotic medication. Estimates of premorbid intelligence, using the National Adult Reading Test (Nelson, 1982), indicated that all schizophrenic subjects were of at least average intelligence before any cognitive decline induced by their illness. The groups did not differ with respect to age, but there were significantly more men than women in the schizophrenic group.

Measures of language expression were not generated in this study, but measures of language comprehension were – specifically, measures for the comprehension of syntax, using a special adaptation of the original token test (de Renzi & Vignolo, 1962).

In the Hobart study discussed before, measures of language comprehension were also recorded. A special version of the token test was also devised for that study, with the introduction of a final part containing syntactically more complex commands (Morice & McNicol, 1985). For the combined groups, as mentioned above, both the total scores on the token test and the final part scores correlated significantly with the derived scores for linguistic performance, at $r = 0.58$ and $r = 0.60$ respectively, both significant at the 0.1% level (Table 5.2). These results have been taken to indicate that similar variants of the token test could be used as reasonable replacement measures of overall linguistic performance, reflecting the degree of syntactic complexity that could be expressed or comprehended while free from syntactic or semantic errors.

In the recent study of executive impairments, a new 50-item version of the token test was used (Morice & Delahunty, unpublished). It comprised ten sections, each of five commands, and with three levels of sentence length, comprised of simple and complex sentences, the complex sentences being divided into right-branching and left-branching sentences (according to the structure of the syntax tree diagram), and the final section comprising sentences that were both right and left branching. Left-branching sentences are more difficult to process, defying, as they do, the English language principles of end-focus and end-weight (Quirk et al, 1972).

Correlation coefficients for the combined groups for the first level of eight- and nine-word simple, right-branching and left-branching sentences, and for

TABLE 5.4
Correlation coefficients (Pearson's r) between total scores on the token test and measures of executive functioning for schizophrenic and control groups combined (n = 38)

	Cognitive flexibility	Forward planning	Working memory
Simple sentences	−0.18	0.15	0.06
Right-branching sentences	−0.10	0.04	0.17
Left-branching sentences	−0.45*	0.43*	0.61**
Total score on the token test	−0.52**	0.43*	0.77**

*$P<0.01$, **$P<0.001$, one-tailed significance.

the total score on the token test, with the three measures of executive functions, are displayed in Table 5.4. The groups were combined to produce more subjects for the matrix, and because general associations were being sought, rather than specific group associations. Significant correlations were recorded for scores on the left-branching section and for total scores on the token test with each of the measures of executive functioning–cognitive flexibility, forward planning, and working memory. The three executive measures were intercorrelated with moderate strength (Table 5.5). Again, and for similar reasons, the combined groups were used.

A stepwise multiple-regression analysis for the combined groups with the total score on the token test as the dependent variable selected only working memory out of the three executive scores entered. It accounted for 60% of the variance in the total scores on the token test. Forced entry of the scores for cognitive flexibility and forward planning did not add to the amount of variance accounted for. When the regressions were performed separately for each diagnostic group, working memory accounted for 56% of the variance in the schizophrenic group, but only for 16% of the variance in the control group.

Some interesting results were obtained for the sentence groups comprising the first level of sentence length (eight words for the simple sentence group, and nine words each for the right- and left-branching sentence groups). Each group comprised five sentences. No errors were made in any group by any of the control subjects. The mean (s.d.) scores for the schizophrenic group were: simple sentences 4.9 (0.2), right-branching sentences 4.9 (0.2), and left-branching sentences 4.2 (1.3). Measures of working memory accounted

TABLE 5.5
Correlation coefficients (Pearson's r) between measures of executive functioning for schizophrenic and control groups combined (n = 38)

	Cognitive flexibility	Forward planning	Working memory
Cognitive flexibility	1.00		
Forward planning	−0.66**	1.00	
Working memory	−0.69**	0.56**	1.00

**$P<0.001$, one-tailed significance.

for 37% of the variance in left-branching sentence scores, but for only 1% of the variance in right-branching sentence scores, and for none of the variance in simple sentence scores.

These results, although they are to be interpreted with caution owing to the small subject numbers, support the contention that some language impairment in schizophrenia could result from executive dysfunction, especially from an impairment in working memory, rather than from specific language dysfunction similar to that resulting from damage to Broca's and Wernicke's areas. Both linguistic performance and its correlate, the total scores on the modified token test, were impaired in the schizophrenic group, as was the main executive correlate, working memory.

Claims that language impairments in schizophrenia result from executive dysfunction are not new. I ventured this claim a few years ago (Morice, 1986b), and followed this with further speculations at the 1988 Winter Workshop on Schizophrenia at Badgastein (Morice, 1988). There I argued that the processing of syntactically complex sentences involved a form of delayed response, the experimental paradigm used in animal prefrontal cortical research.

In order to process complex sentences, I speculated that each embedded clause would have to be processed, and held in a temporary buffer, or 'push-down stack'. All would then have to be retrieved in order to comprehend the entire sentence. I envisaged this 'buffer' as some form of short-term memory. I would now contend that this 'buffer', and the manipulations involved, could be subsumed under the term 'working memory'.

Baddeley (1986) has defined working memory as "a system for the temporary holding and manipulation of information during the performance of a range of cognitive tasks such as comprehension, learning and reasoning" (p. 34). Several groups now have linked impairment of working memory with disordered language processing, albeit usually in association with comprehension rather than expression (Daneman & Carpenter, 1980; Baddeley *et al*, 1985; Yuill *et al*, 1989, Swanson *et al*, 1989; King & Just, 1991; Shapiro *et al*, 1992; McDonald *et al*, 1992).

There have been several other recent interpretations of language impairment in schizophrenia as being due to executive dysfunction (Kaczmarek, 1987; Barr *et al*, 1989; McGrath, 1991), but none of these have invoked the possible role of working memory.

Language impairments resulting from frontal lobe damage have been described since Broca's famous case of 1861 (Signoret *et al*, 1984). However, it is only in more recent years that prefrontal lobe damage has been linked with language impairments. A range of language and cognitive deficits resulting from both medial and dorsolateral prefrontal lesions were reported by Wallesch *et al* (1983). Kaczmarek (1984) reported reduced syntactic complexity in the spoken language of neurological patients with a lesion in the left dorsolateral prefrontal cortex, but not in patients with lesions in the inferomedial cortex. Novoa & Ardila (1987) reported a range of language impairments in patients with both left and right prefrontal damage, although impairments were greater with left-sided damage.

The links between the prefrontal areas of the brain and executive functions are now fairly well established. Patients with prefrontal damage demonstrate a range of executive dysfunctions, best summarised in books by Luria (1984), Stuss & Benson (1986), Perecman (1987), and Fuster (1988). Working memory is an executive function most recently added to the 'prefrontal list' (Goldman-Rakic, 1991, 1992).

To this matrix of associations should be added recent brain-imaging studies. Ingvar (1983), analysing regional cerebral blood flow, found prefrontal activation with silent reading, and also reduced general blood flow in chronic schizophrenic subjects (Ingvar, 1980). Perhaps most persuasively, Weinberger *et al* (1986) demonstrated reduced activation over the left dorsolateral prefrontal cortex of schizophrenic patients when challenged with an executive task, the Wisconsin card sorting test.

Conclusions

Speech and language impairments exist in a substantial number of people with schizophrenia. Using a variety of language metrics, I have endeavoured to show that the expressive language impairments represent a single dimension rather than a bimodal (or even multimodal) one. I have suggested that a test of language comprehension, with enhancements to measure comprehension of complex syntax, can be used as an acceptable, overall measure of linguistic performance, at least with respect to syntactic complexity and syntactic and semantic errors.

I have purported to show that impairment of linguistic performance in schizophrenia is associated with executive dysfunction, especially with impairment of working memory. Executive dysfunctions, including language impairments, or a dysexecutive syndrome (Baddeley, 1986; Morice & Delahunty, 1994*b*), in schizophrenia are most likely subserved by a dysfunctional prefrontal cortex. I temper this contention somewhat by adding that dysfunctions could occur either in the prefrontal cortex itself (which I favour), or in the course of one or more of its many distributed neural networks.

The inability of many schizophrenic people to use speech and language of appropriate complexity without errors must constrain their communication skills, and their ability to comprehend much everyday spoken and written intercourse. Indeed, it must constrain their ability to think with appropriate complexity and clarity.

Viewing the speech and language impairments as possible executive dysfunctions may have implications for the rehabilitation of people with schizophrenia. My colleague, Ann Delahunty, has developed a 'frontal/

executive' rehabilitation programme, an eight-week modular programme predicated upon prefrontal neural circuitry. Improvements in executive functioning, that is, in cognitive flexibility and forward planning, have already accrued in the schizophrenic subjects who have been through the programme (Morice & Delahunty, 1994a). We have not, as yet, measured working memory and linguistic performance before and after this neurocognitive rehabilitation, but we are optimistic that improvements will be found. We hope that the speech and language of these schizophrenia patients will become both less simple and less chaotic.

References

ANDREASEN, N. C. (1982) There may be a "schizophrenic language". *Behavioural and Brain Sciences*, 5, 588–589.
BADDELEY, A. (1986) *Working Memory*. Oxford: Clarendon Press.
——, LOGIE, R., NIMMO-SMITH, J., et al (1985) Components of fluent reading. *Journal of Memory and Language*, 24, 119–131.
BARR, W. B., BILDER, R. M., GOLDBERG, E., et al (1989) The neuropsychology of schizophrenic speech. *Journal of Communication Disorders*, 22, 327–349.
BERG, E. A. (1948) A simple objective technique for measuring flexibility in thinking. *Journal of General Psychology*, 39, 15–22.
BLEULER, E. (1950) *Dementia Praecox, or The Group of Schizophrenias* (trans. J. Zinkin). New York: International Universities Press.
BROCA, P. (1863) Localisations des fonctions cérébrales – Siège du langage articulé. *Bulletins de la Société d'Anthropologie*, 4, 200–204.
CARPENTER, M. D. (1976) Sensitivity to syntactic structure: good versus poor premorbid schizophrenics. *Journal of Abnormal Psychology*, 85, 41–50.
CHOMSKY, N. (1965) *Aspects of the Theory of Syntax*. Cambridge: MIT Press.
CROW, T. J. (1980) Molecular pathology of schizophrenia: more than one disease process? *British Medical Journal*, 280, 66–68.
DANEMAN, M. & CARPENTER, P. A. (1980) Individual differences in working memory and reading. *Journal of Verbal Learning and Verbal Behavior*, 19, 450–466.
DE RENZI, E. & VIGNOLO, L. A. (1962) The token test: a sensitive test to detect receptive disturbances in aphasics. *Brain*, 85, 665–678.
FRASER, W. I., KING, K. M., THOMAS, P., et al (1986) The diagnosis of schizophrenia by language analysis. *British Journal of Psychiatry*, 148, 275–278.
FUSTER, J. M. (1988) *The Prefrontal Cortex*. New York: Raven Press.
GOLDMAN-RAKIC, P. S. (1991) Prefrontal cortical dysfunction in schizophrenia: the relevance of working memory. In *Psychopathology and the Brain* (eds B. J. Carroll & J. E. Barrett), pp. 1–23. New York: Raven Press.
—— (1992) Working memory and the mind. *Scientific American*, September, 73–79.
HEATON, R. K. (1981) *A Manual for the Wisconsin Card Sorting Test*. Odessa: Psychological Assessment Resources.
INGVAR, D. H. (1980) Abnormal distribution of cerebral activity in chronic schizophrenia: a neurophysiological interpretation. In *Perspectives in Schizophrenia Research* (eds C. Baxter & T. Melnechuk). New York: Raven Press.
—— (1983) Serial aspects of language and speech related to prefrontal cortical activity. *Human Neurobiology*, 2, 177–189.
KACZMAREK, B. L. J. (1984) Neurolinguistic analysis of verbal utterance in patients with focal lesions of frontal lobes. *Brain and Language*, 21, 52–58.

KACZMAREK, B. L. J. (1987) Regulatory function of the frontal lobes: a neurolinguistic perspective. In *The Frontal Lobes Revisited* (ed. E. Perecman), pp. 225–240. New York: IRBN Press.
KING, J. & JUST, M. A. (1991) Individual differences in syntactic processing: the role of working memory. *Journal of Memory and Language*, **30**, 580–602.
KING, K., FRASER, W. I., THOMAS, P., et al (1990) Re-examination of the language of psychotic subjects. *British Journal of Psychiatry*, **156**, 211–215.
KLEIST, K. (1960) Schizophrenic symptoms and cerebral pathology. *Journal of Mental Science*, **106**, 246–255.
KRAEPELIN, E. (1919) *Dementia Praecox and Paraphrenia* (trans. R. M. Barclay). Huntingdon: Robert E. Krieger (1971).
LURIA, A. R. (1984) *The Working Brain*. Harmondsworth: Penguin.
MCDONALD, M. C., JUST, M. A. & CARPENTER, P. A. (1992) Working memory constraints on the processing of syntactic ambiguity. *Cognitive Psychology*, **24**, 56–98.
MCGRATH, J. (1991) Ordering thoughts on thought disorder. *British Journal of Psychiatry*, **158**, 307–316.
MORICE, R. (1986a) The structure, organisation, and use of language in schizophrenia. In *Handbook of Studies on Schizophrenia, Part 1* (eds G. Burrows, T. Norman & G. Rubinstein). Amsterdam: Elsevier.
—— (1986b) Beyond language – speculations on the prefrontal cortex and schizophrenia. *Australian and New Zealand Journal of Psychiatry*, **20**, 7–10.
—— (1988) Are language changes in schizophrenia due to an executive dysfunction of prefrontal cortex? *Schizophrenia Research*, **1**, 194.
—— (1990) Cognitive inflexibility and prefrontal dysfunction in schizophrenia and mania. *British Journal of Psychiatry*, **157**, 50–54.
—— & INGRAM, J. C. L. (1982) Language analysis in schizophrenia: diagnostic implications. *Australian and New Zealand Journal of Psychiatry*, **16**, 11–21.
—— & MCNICOL, D. (1985) The comprehension and production of complex syntax in schizophrenia. *Cortex*, **21**, 567–580.
—— & —— (1986) Language changes in schizophrenia: a limited replication. *Schizophrenia Bulletin*, **12**, 239–251.
—— & DELAHUNTY, A. (1994a) Treatment strategies for the remediation of neurocognitive dysfunction in schizophrenia. In *The Neuropsychology of Schizophrenia* (eds C. Pantelis, H. E. Nelson & T. Barnes). Sussex: Wiley (in press).
—— & —— (1994b) Frontal/executive impairments in schizophrenia: cognitive flexibility, forward planning, working memory. (Submitted.)
NELSON, H. E. (1982) *The National Adult Reading Test (NART)*. Windsor: NFER-Nelson.
NOVOA, O. P. & ARDILA, A. (1987) Linguistic abilities in patients with prefrontal damage. *Brain and Language*, **30**, 206–225.
PERECMAN, E. (ed.) (1987) *The Frontal Lobes Revisited*. New York: IRBN Press.
QUIRK, R., GREENBAUM, S., LEECH, G., et al (1972) *A Grammar of Contemporary English*. London: Longman.
ROCHESTER, S. R., HARRIS, J. & SEEMAN, M. V. (1973) Sentence processing in schizophrenic listeners. *Journal of Abnormal Psychology*, **82**, 350–356.
SHALLICE, T. (1982) Specific impairments of planning. *Philosophical Transactions of the Royal Society of London B*, **298**, 199–209.
SHAPIRO, L. P., MCNAMARA, P., ZURIF, E., et al (1992) Processing complexity and sentence memory: evidence from amnesia. *Brain and Language*, **42**, 431–453.
SIGNORET, J. L., CASTAIGNE, P., LHERMITTE, F., et al (1984) Rediscovery of Leborgne's brain: anatomical description with CT scan. *Brain and Language*, **22**, 303–319.
STUSS, D. T. & BENSON, D. F. (1986) *The Frontal Lobes*. New York: Raven Press.
SWANSON, H. L., COCHRAN, K. F. & EWERS, C. A. (1989) Working memory in skilled and less skilled readers. *Journal of Abnormal Child Psychology*, **17**, 145–156.
THOMAS, P., KING, K. & FRASER, W. I. (1987) Positive and negative symptoms of schizophrenia and linguistic performance. *Acta Psychiatrica Scandinavica*, **76**, 144–151.
——, ——, ——, et al (1990) Linguistic performance in schizophrenia: a comparison of acute and chronic patients. *British Journal of Psychiatry*, **156**, 204–210.

WALLESCH, C. W., KORNHUBER, H. H., KOLLNER, C., et al (1983) Language and cognitive deficits resulting from medial and dorsolateral frontal lobe lesions. *Archiv für Psychiatrie und Nervenkrankheiten*, **233**, 279–296.

WEINBERGER, D. B., BERMAN, K. F. & ZEC, R. F. (1986) Physiological dysfunction of dorsolateral prefrontal cortex in schizophrenia. 1: Regional cerebral blood flow evidence. *Archives of General Psychiatry*, **43**, 114–125.

WERNICKE, C. (1874) *Der Aphasische Symptomencomplex. Eine Psychologische Studie auf Anatomischer Basis*. Breslau: M. Cohn und Weigart.

YUILL, N., OAKHILL, J. & PARKIN, A. (1989) Working memory, comprehension ability and the resolution of text anomaly. *British Journal of Psychology*, **80**, 351–361.

6 Thought, speech and language disorder and semantic memory in schizophrenia

ANN MORTIMER, BRYAN CORRIDAN,
SHAUNA RUDGE, KING KHO, FRANK KELLY,
MICHAEL BRISTOW and JOHN HODGES

Complex and incompletely understood relationships exist between thought, language, and speech. In schizophrenia, the clinical phenomenon of thought disorder probably represents an intricate and heterogeneous abnormality in which disturbances of speech, pragmatics, and cognition are all involved. Clinical thought disorder can nevertheless be inferred only by an assessment of what the patient says, as made explicit by Andreasen's (1987) definition: "Positive formal thought disorder is fluent speech that tends to communicate poorly for a variety of reasons". Its characterisation by the psychiatrist, even if the "variety of reasons" are speculated upon, is not neuropsychologically or linguistically based.

In the study of thought disorder, there could be advantages in neuropsychological or linguistic appraisal of speech output, which may be applied more effectively than clinical impression in the experimental setting since deviance is more clearly defined. Such an approach does assume that speech disorder is subordinate to thought disorder, and perhaps affords some potential for unravelling the contributions of language abnormality and cognitive deficit to this clinical phenomenon.

This chapter reviews some ideas and findings on linguistics, cognition, and thought disorder in schizophrenia. It then describes the authors' own study, which took semantic memory dysfunction as a possible basis for clinical thought disorder.

Linguistic problems and thought disorder

Schizophrenic speech is often difficult to understand. The reasons for this may be mechanical, language related, or both. For instance, dysarthria is common, owing to orofacial dyskinesia, oversedation and slurring, or missing or badly fitting teeth. In addition, speech may be aprosodic, with unnatural tone and rhythm. All these factors may cause difficulties in making out what is being said.

Even when words are articulated and heard clearly, the patient may not appear to make much sense: fluent speech communicates poorly, and thought disorder is inferred. The linguistic phenomenon of 'reduced redundancy', that is, speech which is difficult to understand because the meaningfulness of the context of particular words or phrases is reduced, has been investigated in schizophrenia using the cloze procedure. A speech sample is transcribed and then words deleted regularly (e.g. every fifth word). Raters try to fill in the missing words reasonably accurately while preserving the meaning of the whole. This cannot be done as successfully with the speech of schizophrenic subjects as it can with controls, and this seems to be related to thought disorder (Manschreck et al, 1979; Ragin & Oltmanns, 1987).

The possibility of aphasia as a linguistic determinant of schizophrenic speech abnormalities has been studied extensively, although not often in specific relation to thought disorder. Thought processes, nevertheless, appear important to communication on common sense grounds. A simple scheme for the functions necessary in ordinary conversation could be set out as follows:

(a) understanding what is said
(b) formulating a sensible reply
(c) articulating thoughts into spoken language.

All three require thought processes. This may reach consciousness, perhaps most noticeably during formulation of a reply (b), or it may seem effortless and therefore automatic during speech comprehension (a) and articulation (c). Leaving aside the question of whether thoughts can be truly unconscious, it may be argued that (a) and (c) only become conscious when they are effortful, for instance when conversing in a foreign language. Mental activity is going on during all stages of language function, in the form of conscious verbal thoughts when necessary.

If schizophrenic people were impaired in (a), the comprehension aspect, or (c), the articulatory aspect, they would be described as dysphasic. Although some samples of speech in receptive aphasia are similar to thought-disordered speech (Chaika, 1974), more recent work suggests that the resemblance is not complete (Fromkin, 1975; Cohen et al, 1976; List et al, 1977; Strohner et al, 1978; Andreasen & Grove, 1979; Faber et al, 1983). Differences include the breaking of language rules only in certain situations by schizophrenic subjects; the presence of derailment, relative anomia, and features of poverty in schizophrenia; and a relative lack of severity compared with aphasia. As regards expressive aphasia, the only similarity appears to be the simpler grammatical structure of the language of schizophrenic people, with its paucity of helpful conjunctions between ideas expressed (Morice, 1986). A further difference between schizophrenic and aphasic subjects is one of insight, aphasic people being aware of their difficulties, while schizophrenic people are not; this could suggest that the aphasia-like aspects of schizophrenic speech do differ in origin from those of ordinary aphasia.

Overall, it could be proposed that there is some evidence for abnormality in a hypothetical 'central thinking function' (b) beyond the more purely aphasic abnormalities of impaired comprehension and word finding. Circumstantial support may be adduced from the observation that the Comprehensive Assessment of Symptoms and History scale (CASH; Andreasen, 1987), possibly the most detailed instrument for measuring the nature and degree of thought disorder, includes items having considerable validity as indicators of schizophrenic language disorder, such as overinclusiveness (e.g. 'empty philosophising'), derailment, tangentiality, illogicality, and incoherence, as opposed to items more readily congruent with aspects of asphasic speech.

Thought disorder as a cognitive dysfunction

A parsimonious model of thought disorder would attempt to relate all its clinical components to each other in a unitary fashion. While such a model would ignore the proposal that thought disorder is complex and heterogeneous in aetiology, there is a phenomenological tradition of such attempts. For instance, thought disorder has been conceptualised as the result of 'loosening of associations' (Bleuler, 1950), a loss of continuity in which ideas are strung together in a nonsensical fashion. Similarly, it has been ascribed to 'asyndesis' (Cameron, 1944), an inability to preserve conceptual boundaries accompanied by a conspicuous lack of causal logic. These higher-level psychopathologies are, however, no more than further psychiatric phenomena; like the thought disorder they subsume, they are abstract, rather inexact concepts which at best can be measured only subjectively.

It may be more helpful to attempt to characterise thought disorder in terms of neuropsychological deficits, to formulate specific abnormalities in cognitive function which could in theory give rise to aberrations of thought processes. Given such putative abnormalities, the next stage is to identify a suitable test of the relevant aspect of cognitive function, which can be objectively assessed and quantified more accurately than clinical thought disorder. Ideally, the test should make use of the patient's spoken speech or interpretation of speech. To validate the test against thought processes, scores on it should correlate with clinical ratings of thought disorder (despite their disadvantages), preferably obtained independently. A few studies have a bearing on this issue.

Cutting & Murphy (1988) divided thought disorder into three types. One was 'intrinsic thinking disturbance', or 'dyslogia', that is a lack of logic, which was tested by a similarities test, an overinclusiveness test, a proverbs test, and a syllogism test. The distinction was made between dyslogia and another type of thought disorder, 'dysconversation', a disorder of the way thoughts are expressed, tested by a procedure where one of several statements had to be chosen as the most likely antecedent of a reply. Patients did very badly on the dysconversation task, but the possible effect of the dysconversation task being harder than the dyslogia tasks, so patients did not do as well, was not excluded. Double dissociation between the two sorts of tasks (the existence of patients who did badly on dyslogia but not on dysconversation and vice versa) was not unequivocally demonstrated. There did not appear to be a strong relationship between the degree of clinical thought disorder and test performance. However, Cutting's tests had the considerable advantage of direct involvement of patient's language, a criterion widely disregarded in other studies.

McGrath (1991) proposed an explanatory model of thought disorder based on the behavioural functions of the prefrontal lobe. Damage to this area can lead to failure to execute planned behaviour, failure to monitor behaviour for errors, failure to maintain or to change a frame of reference for behaviours, and failure to sequence behaviours appropriately. All these could occur when the behaviour is talking, and the result could be thought-disordered speech. Various authors have shown differences in the speech of schizophrenic compared with control subjects, which suggests such difficulties are manifest. There are also some parallels between the speech abnormalities of some patients with frontal lobe lesions and some schizophrenic patients. In addition, some schizophrenic patients are impaired on some frontal neuropsychological tasks. However, this does not mean that performance on frontal tests relates directly to language disorder, because frontal tasks are not generally language based.

Liddle (1991) proposed from factor analytic studies that thought disorder, along with inappropriate affect, is part of a 'disorganisation syndrome'. This can be conceptualised neuropsychologically as 'failure to inhibit inappropriate responses', which is believed to be a frontal function, making parallels with McGrath's model. Liddle did find a correlation of scores for disorganisation syndrome with scores on frontal tasks which appeared to measure correct inhibition of inappropriate responses, but once again the tasks used did not make direct demands on language.

Frith (1992) has promised a unifying neuropsychological dysfunction in schizophrenia: failure of 'meta-representation', which is the ability to introspect and represent ourselves and the world internally. Disorder of meta-representation implies disorder of self-awareness. Frith proposes that inability to be aware of the self's actions (self-monitoring, including the generation of willed action) and the intentions and cognitions of others may lead to incoherence of speech (the results of the language-based paradigm of Cohen (1976) may be interpreted in this light). Some evidence suggests that on similar tasks, thought-disordered patients perform more poorly than the non-thought disordered (Harvey, 1985). The concept of meta-representation disorder and the consequences of particular aspects of it are in many ways similar to the proposals of McGrath and Liddle.

George & Neufeld (1985) stated that 'loosening of associations', the psychiatric phenomenon which could subsume thought disorder according to Bleuler, may imply a dysfunction of the network of semantic relations held in long-term memory, and that this network presumably underlies the organisation of verbal communication.

Semantic memory is a component of long-term memory, which contains the permanent representation of knowledge of objects, facts, and concepts, as well as words and their meanings. Semantic memory is what gives meaning to sensory experience. In contrast to episodic memory, it is culturally shared; it is common knowledge that grass is green, for instance. Another difference between episodic and semantic memory is that the latter is not temporally specific, that is, items are not tagged with personal time and place information, unlike, for instance, knowing what you had for breakfast or whom you met on holiday last year. Major constituents of semantic memory are acquired early in life when naming, the basis of language, starts to be learned. Semantic memory equates well with what most people would call knowledge, while episodic memory equates to what most people would call simply memory. In the context of neuropsychological tests, semantic memory is vital for the correct identification and naming of objects, and the understanding and production of written and spoken words. It may be divided into two aspects: firstly, the actual store of representations, and secondly, the function of access to these stored representations and their manipulation. Tests of semantic memory are by definition language-related, increasing the suitability of semantic memory as a candidate for the sort of neuropsychological function which, when disordered, may result in thought and language abnormalities. The concept of semantic memory is not dissimilar from Frith's concept of 'second-order representation' (internalised knowledge of the world and its meanings), upon which meta-representation is based. Semantic memory has not been extensively investigated in schizophrenia.

Study 1

In this study (Tamlyn *et al*, 1992), a group of 60 schizophrenic patients aged 19–68 (mean 44.4) years of a wide range of severity and chronicity were recruited. All met the Research Diagnostic Criteria for schizophrenia. Exclusion criteria included a history of organic brain disease, substance abuse, and head injury. All patients were judged to be of normal premorbid intelligence based on schooling, work record, and an estimate of premorbid IQ. These patients had substantial impairments in certain aspects of long-term memory that were disproportionate to the level of general cognitive decline. We were unable to demonstrate any influence of either neuroleptic or anticholinergic medication on these results.

Semantic memory was assessed using the 'silly sentences test' in which the patient is read 50 sentences, some of which are sensible (e.g. 'rats have teeth') and some of which are not (e.g. 'tractors grow in gardens'). The time taken for the patient to reply 'yes' or 'no' to the 50 statements is recorded as a measure of semantic memory processing time. We found that the schizophrenic subjects took a mean of 5.72 seconds per sentence (range 3.7–18 seconds), while a control group had a mean of 3.5 seconds (range 2.76–4.6 seconds). This was a highly significant difference – even the fastest patient was slower than the average normal person. Of even more interest was the finding that nearly a quarter of the sample made multiple incorrect responses to the statements: normal people do not make more than two. Schizophrenic subjects tended to say that silly sentences were true, and it was noticed that clinically these patients were often thought disordered. For instance, a patient replied 'true' to "Screwdrivers have a profession", saying, "They do have a profession, people use them at work. People have a profession who use them, so they're used".

When the number of semantic errors was correlated with the degree of positive formal thought disorder according to the CASH scale, the coefficient was 0.49 ($P<0.001$, Spearman procedure). On cluster analysis of semantic measures and thought disorder in relation to other cognitive tests and clinical phenomena (Fig. 6.1), we found to our surprise that semantic measures clustered with thought disorder and delusions, rather than appearing in the cognitive test cluster.

One problem with using the 'silly sentences test' is that there is a ceiling effect: most patients do not make semantic errors because the test is fairly easy, thus limiting the range of that variable. It is also known that thought

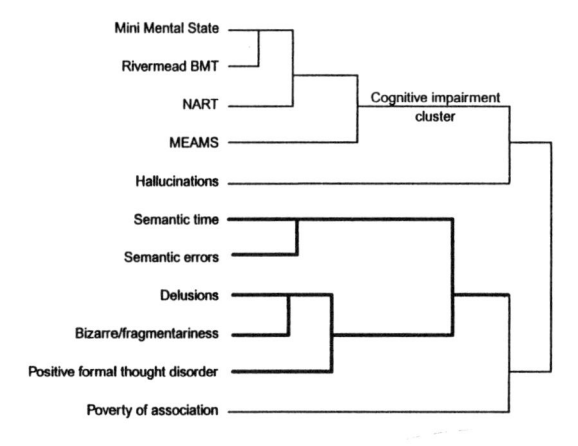

Fig. 6.1. Results of a cluster analysis of cognitive, semantic and clinical ratings among 60 schizophrenic subjects

disorder is most prevalent in acute patients, whereas patients with various chronicities of illness were examined in this study, possibly resulting in similar range restriction for thought disorder. This would tend to detract from the strength of this correlation of 0.49 between the two variables.

Study 2

In order to study the relationship further, 30 patients meeting DSM–III criteria for schizophrenia in acute relapse (age range 23–59 years, mean 34, s.d. 10, mode 25) underwent a detailed assessment of semantic memory less prone to ceiling effects – the Hodges semantic memory battery (Hodges *et al*, 1992). Independent ratings of thought disorder using the CASH were obtained. All patients were of normal premorbid intelligence, as indicated by their completion of normal schooling, and all patients' first language was English. No patient had a history of clinical cognitive impairment of any kind, organic brain disease, or substance abuse.

The Hodges semantic battery

This battery is designed to test semantic knowledge of a carefully matched range of living and man-made items in five different ways, using the same items in each task. Items are depicted by 48 line drawings and represent six semantic categories: land animals (12), sea/water creatures (6), birds (6), household items (12), musical instruments (6), and vehicles (6).

(a) *Fluency*. Patients are given one minute to name exemplars from each semantic category.
(b) *Naming*. Patients are shown 48 line drawings and asked to name items.
(c) *Sorting*.
   Level I. Patients sort line drawings into living versus man-made.
   Level II. Patients sort line drawings into six semantic categories.
   Level III. Patients split land animals, then household items, according to three sets of attributes (e.g. fierce/non-fierce, electrical/non-electrical).
(d) *Word–picture matching*. Patients point to an item asked for by the examiner, choosing it from an array of six items from the same semantic category.
(e) *Generation of definitions*. Patients are given one minute to describe each of 12 items, as if to a person who had never seen one before. The number of statements made is counted, and any perseverations (repeating a statement) and intrusions (incorrect statement, e.g. saying a motorcycle has wings) are also counted.

Tests were administered in the order above.

Results

Thought disorder was strongly correlated with percentage errors on generation of definitions (Spearman correlation coefficient = 0.66, $P<0.001$). There were no other significant associations between test scores (correct, error, and total) and scores for thought disorder.

The performance of the schizophrenic patients on the generation of definitions was compared with that of both a group of Alzheimer patients and a group of matched elderly controls (Hodges *et al*, 1992). Although the total number of statements made by schizophrenic subjects was between that of demented patients and that of elderly controls, their percentage of errors was similar to that of the Alzheimer patients (Fig. 6.2).

No category-specific deficits were observed in any patient or in the patients as a group, either within individual tests or across the whole battery.

Data on three patients were examined for item correspondence between tests (i.e. getting the same items wrong across the five tasks). This may suggest degradation of the semantic store, as described in demented patients, as opposed to failure of access. Only these three patients made mistakes on the word–picture matching task (a total of 21 errors). Eighteen of these 21 items which could not be pointed to were not named correctly either, and none of the items appeared on the patients' fluency lists. Of the total of 38 incorrect names given to items on the naming test by these three patients, 12 appeared on their fluency lists; in contrast, only one correct name

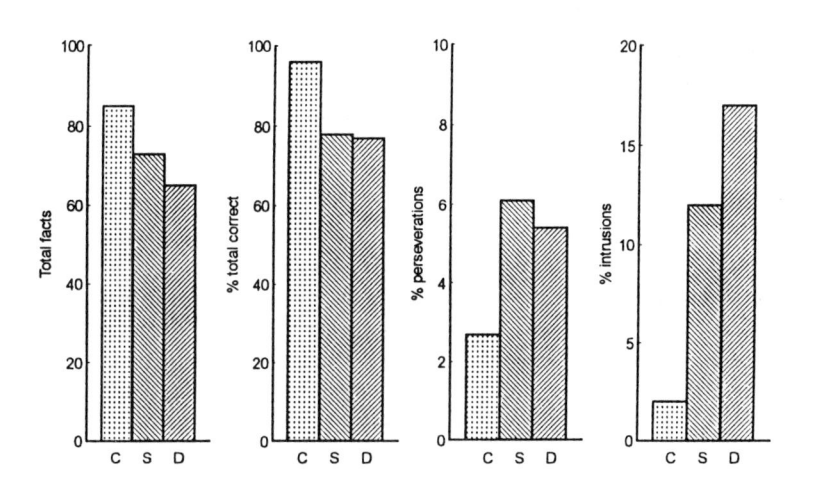

Fig. 6.2. Performance on Hodges generations of definitions of 30 schizophrenic subjects (▨), controls (▦), and patients with Alzheimer's dementia (▧) (data from Hodges et al, 1992)

appeared. On the definitions test, these patients did noticeably worse on items which they could neither point to nor name correctly. As regards thought disorder, two of these patients scored 0 and 1 on the CASH (range 0-25). They made the least and next least number of statements on the definitions test, and their percentage of error statements on the definitions test, 5%, was much smaller than the group mean, of 16%. The third patient had severe thought disorder according to the CASH, and was the fourth worst patient of the 30. Although she, like the other two, made relatively few statements on the definitions test – the 10th fewest of 30 – she was the worst patient at getting them right – 81% of her statements were erroneous.

Discussion

The definitions test is probably the hardest task on the Hodges battery, and it has great face validity as an indication of the use of ordinary language. Therefore its closeness to independently rated thought disorder was striking, and the degree of semantic memory dysfunction implied perhaps renders the severity of schizophrenic language disorder more understandable. These patients seem unable to access their semantic store and its associations correctly. Neither can they manipulate the items; instead they perseverate inappropriately on associations they do access. Such a neuropsychological deficit, reaching the magnitude of that described in demented patients, seems most conspicuous in otherwise healthy young people who have normal premorbid intelligence and no clinical cognitive deficit.

The failure to find category-specific defects argues against a localised lesion (e.g. Pietrini *et al*, 1988) in individual patients or in the patients as a group. This is reasonably consistent with current hypotheses on the pathophysiology of schizophrenia, which do not support the notion of such highly localised abnormalities. It is also consistent with the failure to find prevalent evidence of a deficit of semantic store. However, results on the three exceptional patients suggest item correspondence between the five tests, raising the interesting possibility of a non-category-specific deficit of the semantic store, as described in Alzheimer patients (Hodges *et al*, 1992), in a minority. The absence of correct naming test items on the patients' fluency lists, as opposed to the presence of incorrect names for the same items, suggests that the correct names may have been lost to the patients' semantic store: patients were applying a reduced semantic store inappropriately to the naming task, while many incorrectly named items could not be recognised from an array, even though the name of the item was given. Simply put, these patients were unable to retrieve some items despite several different routes being attempted.

This preliminary evidence for degradation of semantic store is arresting in itself, but how does it relate to the patients' degree of positive thought disorder? In two out of the three patients, it did not – these patients were hardly saying anything, and could be considered to have poverty of thought. This, plus their low scores for positive formal thought disorder, implies that these patients may have isolated problems with their semantic store in the absence of particular semantic access and manipulation difficulties. The third patient, with a high degree of thought disorder and a very high percentage of errors on the definitions test, would appear to have both a disordered semantic store and semantic access/manipulation disorder.

Conclusions

The Hodges definitions test, which taps semantic access and manipulation, is a valid indicator of positive thought disorder, and hence speech and language disorder in schizophrenia.

The majority of patients appear to have problems with semantic access and manipulation, which can reach a level of severity seen in demented patients, while a minority of patients may have semantic store disorder, which may relate to poverty of thought, and hence speech, in schizophrenia.

References

ANDREASEN, N. C. (1987) *The Comprehensive Assessment of Symptoms and History*. Iowa City: University of Iowa College of Medicine.
—— & GROVE, W. (1979) The relationship between schizophrenic language, manic language and aphasia. In *Hemisphere Asymmetries of Function in Psychopathology* (eds J. Gruzelier & P. Flor-Henry). Amsterdam: Elsevier.
BLEULER, E. (1950) *Dementia Praecox, or the Group of Schizophrenias*. New York: International Universities Press.
CAMERON, N. (1944) Experimental analysis of schizophrenic thinking. In *Language and Thought in Schizophrenia* (ed. J. Kasanin). Berkeley: University of California Press.
CHAIKA, E. (1974) A linguist looks at 'schizophrenic' language. *Brain and Language*, **1**, 257–276.
COHEN, B. D. (1976) Referent communication in schizophrenia: the perseverative-chaining model. *Annals of the New York Academy of Sciences*, **270**, 124–141.
COHEN, R., ENGEL, D., KELTER, S., *et al* (1976) Restricted associations in schizophrenics and aphasics. *Archiv für Psychiatrie und Nervenkrankheiten*, **222**, 325–338.
CUTTING, J. & MURPHY, D. (1988) Schizophrenic thought disorder – a psychological and organic interpretation. *British Journal of Psychiatry*, **152**, 310–319.
FABER, R., ABRAMS, R., TAYLOR, M. A., *et al* (1983) Comparison of schizophrenic patients with formal thought disorder and neurologically impaired patients with aphasia. *American Journal of Psychiatry*, **140**, 1348–1351.
FRITH, C. D. (1992) *The Cognitive Neuropsychology of Schizophrenia*. Hove: Lawrence Erlbaum.
FROMKIN, V. A. (1975) A linguist looks at "A linguist looks at 'schizophrenic' language". *Brain and Language*, **2**, 498–503.
GEORGE, L. & NEUFELD, R. J. W. (1985) Cognition and symptomatology in schizophrenia. *Schizophrenia Bulletin*, **11**, 264–285.
HARVEY, P. D. (1985) Reality monitoring in mania and schizophrenia. *Journal of Nervous and Mental Disease*, **173**, 67–73.

HODGES, J. R., SALMON, D. P. & BUTTERS, N. (1992) Semantic memory impairment in Alzheimer's disease: failure of access or degraded knowledge? *Neuropsychologia*, **30**, 301–314.

LIDDLE, P. F. (1991) Schizophrenic syndromes and frontal lobe performance. *British Journal of Psychiatry*, **158**, 340–345.

LIST, G., COHEN, R., ENGEL, D., *et al* (1977) Zum Einfluß von syntaktischer Struktur und Proximitat auf Assoziationen zu Satzteilen bei aphatischen und schizophrenen Patienten. *Zeitschrift für klinische Psychologie*, **6**, 100–115.

MANSCHRECK, T. C., MAHER, B. A., RUCKLOS, M. E., *et al* (1979) The predictability of thought-disordered speech in schizophrenic patients. *British Journal of Psychiatry*, **134**, 595–601.

MCGRATH, J. (1991) Ordering thoughts on thought disorder. *British Journal of Psychiatry*, **158**, 307–316.

MORICE, R. (1986) The structure, organisation and use of language in schizophrenia. In *Handbook of Studies on Schizophrenia. Part I: Epidemiology, Etiology and Clinical Features* (eds G. D. Burrows, T. R. Norman & G. Robinson). Amsterdam: Elsevier.

PIETRINI, V., NERTEMPI, P., VAGLIA, A., *et al* (1988) Recovery from herpes simplex encephalitis: selective impairment of specific semantic categories with neuroradiological correlation. *Journal of Neurology, Neurosurgery and Psychiatry*, **51**, 1284–1293.

RAGIN, A. B. & OLTMANNS, T. F. (1987) Communicability and thought disorder in schizophrenics and other diagnostic groups. *British Journal of Psychiatry*, **154**, 52–57.

STROHNER, H., COHEN, R., KELTER, S., *et al* (1978) "Semantic" and "acoustic" errors of aphasic and schizophrenic patients in a sound–picture matching task. *Cortex*, **14**, 391–403.

TAMLYN, D., MCKENNA, P. J., MORTIMER, A. M., *et al* (1992) Memory impairment in schizophrenia – its extent, affiliations and neuropsychological character. *Psychological Medicine*, **2**, 101–115.

7 Schizophasia: the glossomanic and the glossolalic subtypes

ANDRÉ ROCH LECOURS

The word 'schizophrenia' was coined by Bleuler (1911) to describe a family of thought disorders, fundamental manifestations of which, it was later found, remain constant irrespective of epochs and societies (Cancro, 1983). This has led many to suggest that schizophrenia is indeed a single nosological entity, and to suspect that it stems, at least in part, from organic causes (Weiner, 1983).

Given the ability to speak, thought disorders are bound to express themselves in speech (among other behaviours). Clinicians agree that certain speech behaviours can readily be recognised as manifestations of schizophrenia, but the diagnosis of schizophrenia on the basis of schizophrenic speech depends on a largely overlapping and impressionistic terminology. The following list, borrowed to a large extent from Andreasen (1979a), is not exhaustive: 'poverty of speech', 'laconic speech', 'poverty of content of speech', 'poverty of thought', 'empty speech', 'alogia', 'verbigeration', 'negative formal thought', 'pressure of speech', 'distractible speech', 'tangentiality', 'derailment', 'loose associations', 'paralogia', 'flight of ideas', 'incoherence', 'illogicality', 'clanging', 'neologisms', 'word approximations', 'metonyms', 'circumstantiality', 'loss of goal', 'perseveration', 'echolalia', 'blocking', 'stilted speech', 'self-reference', 'word salad'.

Given the richness and diversity of this lexicon, it does not come as a surprise that the single nosological entity known as schizophrenia encompasses, according to Andreasen (1979b), no less than 18 subtypes of thought disorder, one of which is 'poverty of content of speech'. It is illustrated by the following quotation:

> "Many of the problems that I have . . . are difficult for me to handle or to work on because I am not aware of them as problems which upset me personally. I have to get my feelers way out to see how it is . . . I am, I think, becoming more aware that perhaps, on an analogy, the matter of some who understand or enjoy loud rages of anger. . . . The same thing can be true for other people and I have to kind of try to learn to see when that is true and what I can do about it."

It has been suggested that 'schizophrenic speech' of this type is somehow similar to the discourse of certain aphasic people (Chaika, 1974). Consider, for instance, the following excerpt from a tape-recorded conversation with a right-handed male patient who showed evidence of transcortical sensory aphasia as the result of a left inferior parietal stroke (Lecours et al, 1981a):

> "C'est assez compliqué, hein. Ça devient assez compliqué de . . . de tirer ça[1] . . . . 'J'arrive à faire que le total arrive à faire un certain bien . . . et qu'on arrive à arriver à . . . à avoir des . . . des marchandises."
>
> "It is quite complicated, eh. It becomes quite complicated to . . . to make this. . . . I manage to do that the total manages to do something good . . . and that we manage to manage to . . . to have some . . . some merchandises."

Although comparable with regard to phonological and to syntactic procedures, the two samples above are fundamentally different: the first is lexically rich and the second is not. If Andreasen's quotation is indeed illustrative of what is clinically labelled as 'poverty of content of speech', it might be that this type of speech behaviour would be better qualified as a verbal interaction in which communication remains poor, conceivably because one of the protagonists' language does not represent conventional thought (but this goes beyond the topic of this chapter).

According to Porot (1975), the word 'schizophasia' was coined by Kraepelin. To the best of my knowledge, and beyond the fact that this label also stands for episodic behaviours coexisting with conventional speech abilities, there is no convincing documentary evidence that might lead one to take it as a synonym for 'schizophrenic speech'. Indeed, I am not certain that only schizophrenic people are capable of 'schizophasia', although, unless otherwise specified, all of the examples below are from individuals who were diagnosed schizophrenic.

The term 'schizophasia' designates, specifically, at least two forms of unconventional surface speech behaviours – 'glossomanic behaviour' and 'glossolalic behaviour' – which can be observed in certain psychotic patients (Lecours et al, 1981b). Both can be spectacular, but neither is now a frequent clinical phenomenon, perhaps because of the modern use of potent drugs.

The essential characteristic of 'glossomanic schizophasia' is the production of utterances the linguistic components of which – be they phonemes, words, or more complex units – are selected and combined on the basis of superficial or semantic kinships rather than by compliance to an immediately sharable topic. The main characteristics of 'glossolalic schizophasia' is an entirely or nearly entirely neologistic discourse.

---

1. Probably "tirer ça au clair", that is, "to make this clear".

A simple model of speech

It would be useful first to summarise, by reference to a naïve model (or 'functional architecture'), some of the prerequisites of speech, whether conventional or not (Fig. 7.1).

Speech behaviour is triggered by an intention, and this intention is modulated, at least in part, by one's affect (hence the two 'clouds' in the upper part of Fig. 7.1).

Unless speech is governed only by one's knowledge of the learned conventions of 'phonological procedures' and of 'morphological and syntactic procedures' (see below), it could not take place without some conceptual knowledge of oneself and one's environment. This conceptual stock is identified here as the *Begriffsvermögen*. Neither could speech take place without memories of spoken words as they are decoded and encoded. These particular 'bins' are identified in Fig. 7.1 as the input and output logophonic lexicons.

If speech is governed only by one's knowledge of the learned conventions of rule-governed phonological procedures, that is, if both the *Begriffsvermögen* and the logophonic lexicons are turned off, then speech can take place only if 'stocks' of sublexical units are available, both in their auditory and in their kinaesthetic forms. It is postulated here that these sublexical units are syllables (Bertelson, 1986; Bertelson *et al*, 1987; Bertelson & de Gelder, 1989; Mann, 1986; Morais *et al*, 1979, 1986; Read *et al*, 1986), hence the designation of the corresponding stores as the input and output 'phonosyllabic registers'.

In all cases, the interactions between any two stocks are postulated to be specifically mediated by various 'access', 'matching', or conversion procedures'. These procedures also pertain to the domain of memory.

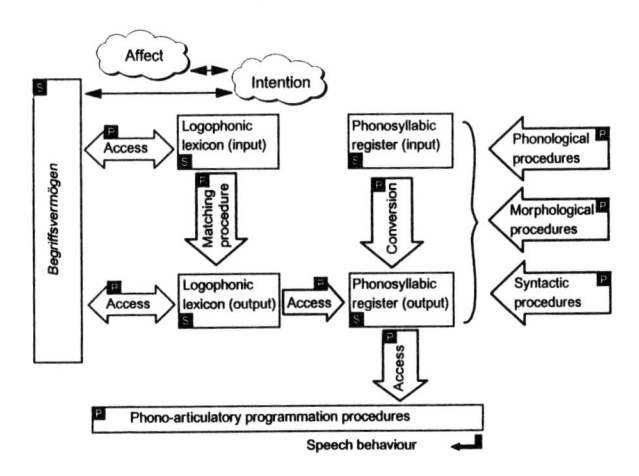

Fig. 7.1. A general model of speech and its prerequisites

In Fig. 7.1, each white 'S' on a black square identifies a specialised memory of the stock type, that is, a particular bin of learned information, such as the mental representations of input words or those of output syllables. Each white 'P' on a black square identifies a memorised procedure specific to the interactions between two given bins. The figure represents a direct metaphor of mind rather than of brain function. Indirectly, it can also be taken as potential metaphors for anatomical, histological, or chemical substrata.

Glossomanic schizophasia

Glossomanic schizophasia is a particular form of fluent speech. Just as with the prototype of Wernicke's jargon aphasia, it requires only minimal participation from the interlocutor. It comprises occasional word-like but neologistic entities of three different types: derived morphemic deviations; composed morphemic deviations; and abstruse neologisms (Lecours & Vanier-Clément, 1976; Lecours, 1982*a*).

Derived morphemic deviations

These are morphologically constrained word-like entities. The speaker associates legitimate roots and bound morphemes in line with the word-derivation rules inherent in the language, thereby creating neologisms. Here are a few examples:

Prefix +	*page* + suffix (pageboy)	→	*apagé* (one who is being made a pageboy)
Prefix +	*page* + suffix (pageboy)	→	*apageant* (one who makes someone else a pageboy)
Prefix +	*page* + suffix (pageboy)	→	*apagement* (the fact of being made a pageboy)
Prefix +	*capitale* (capital city)	→	*acapitale* (without a capital city)
douane + (custom)	suffix	→	*douanerie* (custom system)
logarithme + (logarithm)	suffix	→	*logarithmie* (logarithmic system)

In the first of these examples, the patient adds the legitimate prefix [a] and legitimate suffix [e] to a root, [paʒ], meaning either 'pageboy' or 'page of a book', therefore creating a neologism that potentially represents 'one who is being made a pageboy'. (The three neologisms would of course have different meanings if *page* is taken as 'page of a book'.)

Composed morphemic deviations

These are lexically – as opposed to morphologically – constrained. The speaker now associates at least two legitimate words in line with the word composition rules of the language, thereby creating a second form of neologism. The following examples were produced by the same patient who entertained thoughts about pageboys (or pages of books).

quart	+ *cinquième*	→	*quart-cinquième*
(quarter)	(fifth)	→	(quarter-fifth)
été	+ *hiver*	→	*été-hiver*
(summer)	(winter)	→	(summer-winter)
jour	+ *nuit*	→	*jour-nuit*
(day)	(night)	→	(day-night)
ouvre	+ *ferme*	→	*ouvre-ferme*
(open)	(close)	→	(open-close)

It is common, in this form of glossomania, for a neologism to be created by associating antonymic roots, as is the case in each of the last three examples above.[2] This type of production is a manifestation of Laffal's 'opposite speech' (Porot, 1975). A more elaborate form is illustrated by the same subject when he utters:

"Un bureau ambulant, un cadavre vivant, où . . ."

"A perambulating office, a living corpse, where . . ."

'Opposite speech' ('antonymy') is often a spectacular schizophasic behaviour. It is also a variety of 'tangentiality' (Andreasen, 1979a), as schizophasic individuals also play on words that are not counterparts. For instance, as shown below, one can create a formally valid but whimsical utterance linking 'human' to 'physique', then to 'animal' to 'vegetable', and to 'star':

"c'est-à-dire que le physique humain, euh . . . animal et végétal, est classé d'abord, naturellement, par l'astre, et l'humain classe l'astre également."

"that is to say that the human physique, hem . . . the animal and the vegetable, is first of all classified, naturally, by the star, and the human also classifies the star."

---

2. If one agrees with Freud's (1910) teachings on the relationships between negation, dreaming, and what he calls the "primal words" of humanity, one might surmise that the species was born schizophrenic.

Abstruse neologisms

As in the two examples below, the speaker typically borrows sounds from the immediate context in order to create a word-like entity.

> "Je fais mon classement des [sudɔʃʀi] d'où je viens. . . . C'est pestilentiel, vous savez, cette soude [sud] . . . du duché [dyʃe] ou de communale."
>
> "I make my classification of the [sudɔʃʀi] from where I come. . . . It stinks, you know, this soda . . . of the dukedom or commune."
>
> "en perdant la maîtrise de sa classification, en allant dire des grossièretés [gʀosjɛʀte]. . . . C'est une espèce de maladie, de [gʀosjomiʒ]."
>
> "by loosing the mastery of one's classification, by being gross in speech. . . . It is a kind of disease, of [gʀosjomiʒ]."

In the first example, the speaker borrows from the French for soda [sud] and dukedoms [dyʃe] to produce *'soudocherie'*. In the second, he creates *'grossiomige'*, in which he adds or perhaps subtracts something to the notion of 'gross speech' [gʀosjɛʀte].

Bleuler (1911) wrote that some psychotic patients will discuss the meaning of their abstruse neologisms, if asked to do so. *'Grossiomige'* turned out to be a 'personal' and 'private' 'beast'.

> "Oui. C'est une espèce de bête. Voilà! C'est un terme que j'ai créé, que j'ai fait, comme ça, pour . . . pour donner une petite base personnelle, privée. Voilà."
>
> "Yes. It is a kind of beast. That's it! It is a word that I have created, that I have made, like that, to . . . to provide a small, personal and private basis. That's it!"

I have never observed this phenomenon in Wernicke's jargon aphasia.

Glossomanic utterances

Glossomanic utterances are phrases including some of the ingredients that have been defined above. Sometimes the utterances comprise words with a phonological kinship:

> "C'est comme ça que les vieux faisaient les fondations. Ou bien de cause [koz]: un [kozam], un [klozam], [glozan]. Vous comprenez? Et, à ce casier, on a un savoir de Lausanne [lozan]."
>
> "It is this way that the ancient built foundations. Or else of cause: a [kozam], a [klozam], [glozan]. You understand? And, in this bin, one has a knowledge from Lausanne."

In this example, a syntactically acceptable utterance brings together five phonological congeners. The first is a legitimate word, [koz]. The next three are abstruse neologisms: [kozam], [klozam], and [glozam] (to cause or to speak, to close, and to gloss, perhaps). The last, [lozan], is the name of the city where the patient was interviewed.

The following example is from Chaika's (1974) first publication on this topic. Her patient also produced a syntactically valid utterance, this time founded on semantic kinships: Saint Valentine is linked to breeding and, thereafter, to birds, to buzzards, and to parakeets, all of which are cooing creatures:

> "My mother's name was Bill . . . and coo? St Valentine's Day is the official startin' of the bredin' season of the birds. All buzzards can coo. I like to see it pronounced buzzards rightly. They work hard. So do parakeets."

Glossomanic speakers usually resort to both phonological and semantic kinships, independently or jointly. In the example below, the man from Lausanne plays with the phonological French kinship between 'cheeks', 'days', and the act of 'opening': *joues, jours, ouvrir*. He also plays with the antonymy between the notions of opening and closing, and with the French homononyms for 'to close' and 'country farm' (*ferme*):

> "Et alors, il y a des joues, [ʒu], jours [ʒuR], des j'ouvre-ferme [ʒuvR-fɛRm] qui sont des fermes [fɛRm] de campagne."

> "And then, there are some cheeks, days, some I open-close which are country farms."

In the next example, the same patient gathers the semantics of time and weather: calendar goes with clock, minutes, and hours, and also with storm and thunder. He also gathers sounds, in several manners. For instance *'heure'* [œR] and *'or'* [ɔR] are put together: the hour and the gold. The net result is incomprehensible at first sight:

> "Mais oui, à cette organisation de travail, il y a donc des plans d'heures [œR] et un calendrier du plan de secondes, de minutes, d'heures [œR], d'horlogerie [ɔRlɔʒRi] et d'orage (or-âge) [ɔR-aʒ]. Vous appelez ça des heures-âges [œR-aʒ], d'où des tonnages (tonnes-âges) [tɔn-aʒ] qui, de l'âge [aʒ] du début d'un certain âge [aʒ], par rapport au calendrier . . ."

> "Yes indeed, to this organisation of work, there are thus draughts of hours and a calendar of the draught of seconds, of minutes, of hours, of clock-making and of orage. You call that hour-ages, hence ton-ages which, from the age of the beginning of a certain age, by reference to the calendar . . ."

I shall quote a few further illustrative examples. Three are from Lausanne and three are from Levy-Valensi *et al* (1931): the first two illustrate the speaker's limited although creative potential for adding a few tricks to his automated phonological procedures; the third is a masterpiece of free, although rule-governed, morphology; and the last three illustrate how one can transform clauses and sentences into single lexical units.

The first two examples illustrate deliberate phonological transgression (a phenomenon which is never observed in aphasia). The man from Lausanne invents, explains, and applies rules leading him to the production of a few neologisms, two of which – [pRɔRʃ] in the first quotation, [ʧʃowa] and [fRʃowa] in the second – are not legitimate in standard French:

> "Si vous marchez, vous allez comme ceci: c'est un classement de pas. Et, à l'origine, le vieux dialecte. . . . C'est un [pRa] et non pas un pas. Pourquoi un [pRa]? Parce que 'P' onomatopique-hiéroglyphique est à 'R'. Il est à 'R': un [pRa]. Pourquoi un [pRa]? Parce que euh les . . . les . . . les définitions du nom . . . des noms furent faites ainsi, pour le laïque, l'ecclésiastique. . . . Alors, on marche à [pRa], de [pRɔʃ] et de [pRɔʃ]. . . . Vous comprenez?"

> "If you walk, you go like this: it is a step classification. And, at the origin, the old dialect. . . . It is a 'strep', and not a step. Why a 'strep'? Because the onomatopoeic-hieroglyphic 'P' relates to 'R'. It relates to 'R': a 'strep'. Why a 'strep'? Because hem the . . . the . . . the definitions of the name . . . of the names were thus made, for the layman, the ecclesiastic. . . . Therefore, one walks by 'strep', from 'nrear' and from 'nrear'. . . . You understand?"

The phonologically illegitimate non-word in this quotation potentially associates the notion of walking and of getting where you wish to go. In the second quotation, it is an explicit concatenation of hot and cold:

> "De froid-chaud ou de chaud-froid. De [ʧʃoWa]. Ils. . . . Ils parlaient comme ça, les anciens. Ils disaient un [ʧʃRowa]. C'était les anciens qui parlaient ainsi."

> "Of cold-hot or of hot-cold. Of 'cohotld'. They. . . . They talked like that, the ancients. They said a 'cohotld'. It was the ancients who talked like that."

Now let us consider free morphology:

> "Pour prendre une pierre, ils l'appelèrent une pierre . . . la lever et la poser. Ils 'dépierrent' à 'repierrer', n'est-ce-pas? C'est juste. Et on les appela 'dépierrarepierra'. On les appela les roches de la roche, de définition. Et ils 'arrochent' des roches. Vous comprenez? Et les deux pierres à deux roches, ça devient des 'procha'. A classement de . . . de généralité (n'est-ce pas?), transpositif de 'pierra' est à 'rocha'. 'Rocha' est à . . . est à deux 'pierra' mais, à la synthèse des deux, c'est un 'procha de pierra' ou 'de rocha'."

> "To take a stone, they named it a stone . . . to lift it up and to put it down. They 'unstone' to 'restore', is it not? It is fair. And they were named unstoned-restoned. They were named the rocks of the rocks, by definition. And they 'arock' some rocks. You understand? And the two stones to two rocks, they became 'strocka'. In a classification of . . . of generality (is it not?), transpositive

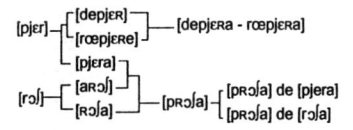

```
                    ┌─[depjɛR]──┐
        ┌─[depjɛR]──┤           ├─[depjɛRa - rœpjɛRa]
[pjɛr]──┤  [rœpjɛRe]│
        └─[pjɛra]───┘
                    ┌─[aRɔʃ]────┐              ┌─[pRɔʃa] de [pjɛra]
[rɔʃ]───┤           │           ├─[pRɔʃa]──────┤
        └─[Rɔʃa]────┘              └─[pRɔʃa] de [rɔʃa]
```

Fig. 7.2. 'Mirror derivation' of two neologisms, stemming from 'pierre' (stone) and 'roche' (rock)

of 'stona' is to 'rocka'. 'Rocka' is to . . . is to two 'stona' but, at the synthesis of the two, it is a 'strocka of stona' or 'of rocka'.''

This formally coherent set of consecutive sentences is founded, essentially, on a mirror derivational overuse of two synomic roots, that is 'stone' and 'rock' (*pierre* [pjɛR] and *roche* [Rɔʃ]) (Fig. 7.2). 'Stone' comes first, then 'unstone' and 'restone', followed by 'unstoned-restoned'. 'Rock' comes second, and it engenders 'arock'. The ground is thereafter ready for root blending: thus enters a new pair of synonyms, neologistic ones this time: 'strocka of stona' and 'strocka of rocka'. The transcript shown in Fig. 7.2 represents the mirror derivation.

I have only once observed in Wernicke's jargon aphasia (in a right-handed man with left temporal brain damage) a significant number of neologisms which qualified as derived 'morphemic deviations' (Lecours & Lhermitte, 1972). The patient was a general of the French army, he had written several books on military tactics, and his neologistic derivations were somewhat poor and perseverative. On the other hand, it is well documented that the abstruse neologisms of Wernicke's aphasics often end on a conventional suffix (Buckingham & Kertesz, 1976).

In the examples from Levy-Valensi *et al* (1931) ''subdue me'', ''the soul is weary'', and ''so beautiful is the area that one has to raise it up with facts'' all have become expanded words, or compacted sentences:

''Je fais de l'âme est lasse à toujours vous servir . . .''

''I make some the soul is weary as I always serve you . . .''

''Si vous voulez faire le tant l'aire est belle qu'il la faut majorer de faits, c'est que vous êtes . . .''

''If you wish to make the so beautiful is the area that one has to raise it up with facts, it is because you are . . .''

''. . . faire un beau maîtrisez moi.''

''. . . to make a beautiful subdue me.''

These samples were written (schizographic), not spoken (schizophasic).

The glossomanic schizophasic is one who is more easily taken at her/his words (or word-like creations) rather than – as convention suggests – at her/his phrases.

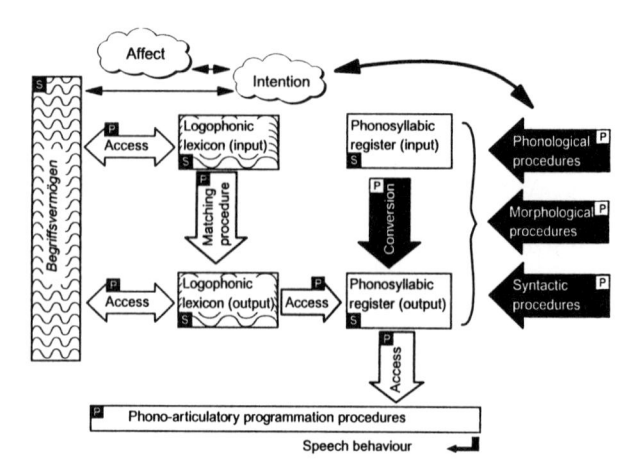

Fig. 7.3. A model of glossomanic schizophrenia

Figure 7.3 represents glossomanic schizophrenia. On the left side, the *Begriffsvermögen* is filled with 'waves' which do not hamper the speaker's ability to recognise semantic kinships between words, but which are strong enough to hide the speaker's message (if there is any). This is not the case in 'poverty of content of speech'. There are also 'waves' in the lexicons, which apparently favour recognition of superficial kinships between words, whether or not these are conceptually related. On the right side of Fig. 7.3 there is formidable overuse of phonological, morphological, and syntactic procedures. Phonological hyperactivity permits the creation of new conversion rules, hence the blackened arrow between the 'registers'.

Glossomanic schizophrenia might be defined as a cleverly built discourse in which words and word-like entities are associated in view of their superficial and semantic kinships rather than in the function of a conventional topic to be communicated. This behaviour would qualify as a form of hyperphasia, not unlike that of certain precocious children, nor, for that matter, unlike that of certain poets.

Glossolalic schizophasia

'Glossolalia' (Cénac, 1925) was defined above as an entirely or nearly entirely neologistic discourse. Some people enjoy doing it when possessed by gods (Samarin, 1972) or demons, some will do it on demand, usually to their own surprise (Lecours, 1982*b*), and some well-known poets also use it (Antonin Artaud, for instance).

Glossolalia can also (rarely) be the single residual speech ability left in certain cases of Wernicke's jargon aphasia. I have observed one case only, that of a bilingual elderly retired man who enjoyed writing poetry before his stroke (Lecours *et al*, 1981*a*).

Some psychotic people will produce glossolalic schizophasia for hours, and then revert to conventional speech (which no aphasic person can do). Bobon (1947), for instance, has reported the case of a patient who could speak what his psychiatrist qualified as "three artificial tongues of ludic origin". Bobon's diagnosis for this patient was hypomanic paraphrenia. I have observed, recorded and transcribed only one psychotic subject (GL) who episodically switched to glossolalic discourse, and this subject could also speak three artificial tongues (Lecours, 1982*b*). GL respectively identified each of his three tongues as his 'English temper', his 'French temper', and his 'funny temper'. Although poorly educated and a unilingual speaker of East Montreal French, GL somehow managed to make his English temper sound like a regular Spanish-like paroxytone. His French temper shared the tonic accent of standard French, and it permitted the use of three or four closed-class words, as well as that of a comparable number of suffix-like entities. The tonic accent of his (more recent) funny temper was far less predictable. None of GL's three tempers resorted to unconventional phonology.

As a peace-time private in the Canadian army, GL enjoyed listening – at length – to foreign radio broadcasts of various origins. He claimed that he had once worked as a 'crooner' on Mars. He insisted that his glossolalic utterances were dictated directly into his head by an external will, and that he should therefore be considered as a mere transmission instrument. GL's psychiatrist considered his patient's condition to be prototypical schizophrenia.

If GL is representative, as I think he is, glossolalic schizophasia takes the form of asemantic, although prosodically invested, monologues, in which the tonic accent of a unilingual speaker's mother tongue can be replaced by another. I might add that the speaker's regional accent can be erased, or nearly so (as often happens when people sing). Phonemes are those of the mother tongue, but their relative frequencies are grossly modified (phonemes that are relatively infrequent in standard speech can be overused and vice versa, and certain phonemes are totally absent from given samples).

Jargonaphasic glossolalia is quite different, not only because it is a residual behaviour, but also because it occurs only within dialogue, because prosody and accent remain those of the subject's premorbid conversational habits, and also because phonemic frequencies remain somewhat closer to norms (no sound is systematically excluded and systematic overuse is less striking, although perseverative components are present).

If one listens to glossolalic speech, or else if one ponders on transcripts, one often remains under the impression that it is made of word-like and sentence-like entities. It might be that this impression depends, to some extent, on prosodic factors. Documenting one's impression beyond prosody is an altogether different matter. One must first accept the notion that glossolalic speakers memorise word-like entities without a socially sharable meaning. With specific regard to his English temper, GL did just that with ten items, each with its own variants: (1) [azúmba], (2) [bergés], (3a) [kóro], (3b) [kerœkóru], (4) [brubjér], (5) [pára], (6) [brázje mnerges], (7) [arakáska rœkárœ], (8a) [mísi], and (8b) [mízœ príz]. Each variant was the result of one or two vowel changes. For instance, item 3b in this list, [kerœkóru], could mutate into [kerokúru]. My supposition is that this was due to a certain instability in the corresponding mental representations of these word-like units in GL's self-made 'English temper' lexicon. However, such variants might have been the expression of a superfluous automated mental procedure (perhaps even of a deliberate one). When I told GL that his English temper words were few and repetitive, he agreed, somewhat reluctantly, and retorted at once that, if the number of these words was indeed small, their meanings could differ widely from one context to another. He added that he, himself, did not understand them, since they were dictated to him by a foreign mind; and also that I, as a scientist, should be able to decode them appropriately.

These word-like entities could be combined in a rule-governed manner, that is, in line with a 'grammar'. All of the sentence-like utterances in an uninterrupted 15-minute sample abided by the combination rules summarised below. This grammar first recognises the legitimacy of three clauses. Two of these ('A' and 'B') include the other ('a'):

a = (3a or 3b + 4)
A = (5 + 6 + a)
B = (8b + 7 + 6 + a)

All of GL's English temper 'sentences' abided by a single rule:

$$1 \pm 2 + a + \left| \begin{array}{c} A \\ or \\ B \end{array} \right| \pm A + \left| \begin{array}{c} 8 \\ or \\ (B + 8) \\ or \\ (B + B + 8) \\ or \\ (B - 4) \end{array} \right|$$

This grammar is very simple, as was GL's French temper. The same is true of charismatic (religious) glossolalia. On the other hand, no grammar could be documented in GL's 'funny temper', and neither in a lengthy transcript from a case of Wernicke's glossolalia, nor in a long poetic trancript. This leads to the supposition that the latter samples might have played exclusively on phonology.

My assumptions concerning glossolalia, schizophasic or otherwise, are summarised in Fig. 7.4. On the left side of the graph, the *Begriffsvermögen* is

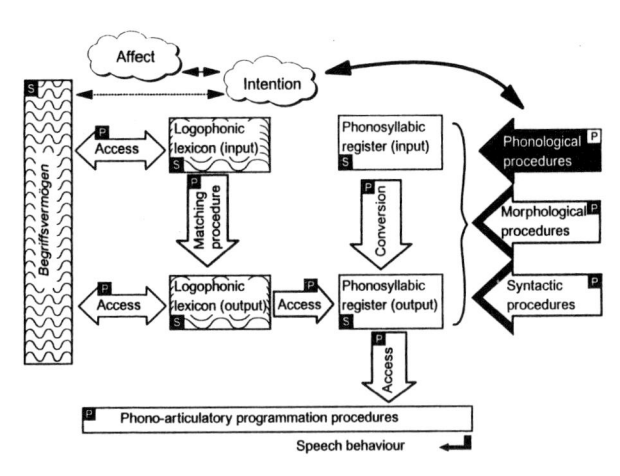

Fig. 7.4. A model of glossolalic schizophasia

again filled with 'waves', which are apparently strong enough to turn it off. The difference between schizophasic and aphasic glossolalia, in this respect, is that the *Begriffsvergmögen* is turned off temporarily in the former, that is, as long as the speaker wishes it or is bound to 'glossolalise', whereas it is turned off permanently in the latter. The black arrow on the right side suggests that there are cases in which exploitation of learned 'phonological procedures' is the only mechanism on which glossolalic discourse depends. In such cases, the waves in the lexicons thus indicate that these components are also turned off, temporarily or permanently, depending on whether or not glossolalic behaviour is the result of acquired brain damage. The two blackened arrowheads on the right side suggest that there are also cases in which limited use of 'morphosyntactic' procedures has become possible with practice. As far as it is known, this is not possible in aphasia resulting from brain damage; the lexicons are also turned off in such cases, with the exception of a few neologistic although memorised word-like entities. GL's English temper may be taken as evidence of this.

The glossolalic schizophasic is one who should first be taken at his/her phonemes, or syllables. By comparison to glossomania, glossolalia might be conceived as an 'underfed hyperphasia'. Syllabic memories are impoverished, but they are, nevertheless, overexploited, a few particularly so.

Beyond that, there are cases in which glossolalic phonological routines engender a tiny lexicon of word-like units, and in which these are in turn used following the rules of a minimal grammar. It should be noted that the former is far smaller than that of a standard dolphin, and that the latter goes far past any chimpanzee's innate abilities. (The case of Hélène Smith remains an exception (Flournoy, 1900).)

Conclusions

Glossomanic schizophasia can share certain linguistic features with one form or another of fluent aphasia but, whereas evidence of partial or complete loss of at least one and usually several of the stocks and procedures behind language production is always manifest in the latter, it is evidence of procedural hyperfunction – for instance, exaggerated but accurate use of word-derivation rules – that dominates glossomania. Whether or not glossomanic schizophasia should always be considered as a manifestation of schizophrenia or that of another form of psychosis remains an open question. Glossomanic schizophasics can give proof of such mastery of rule-governed language that one can hardly conceive of their behaviour as being a manifestation of acquired focal brain damage. The main difference between spectacular glossomania and certain forms of literary creation is that the first appears to be exclusively founded on phonological and/or semantic kinships between words, whereas the second is both founded on such kinships and is guided by topic.

Although glossolalia is uncommon in aphasia and has so far been observed exclusively in brain-damaged polyglot elderly people, glossolalic jargon can occur as a form of Wernicke's aphasia. This condition and glossolalic schizophasia are similar if one considers them exclusively from the phonological point of view. None the less, they differ in that the latter represents residual behaviour, takes the form of a dialogue with an interlocutor, and retains conversational prosody, whereas the glossolalia of schizophrenic subjects occurs episodically (i.e. coexists with a capacity for conventional speech), is produced as monologues, and mimics one form or another of stereotyped prosody. The two also differ in that schizophasic but not jargonaphasic glossolalia resorts to limited 'neo-lexical' stocks and still more limited morphosyntactic procedures.

Finally, the semantic dysfunction is strong enough to turn off the *Begriffsvermögen* in glossolalic schizophasia, and strong enough to limit its function to root-kinships recognition in glossomanic schizophasia, whereas it might be a vastly more subtle conceptual dysfunction that expresses itself through the discourse of those considered to show evidence of schizophrenic speech.

References

ANDREASEN, N. J. C. (1979a) Thought, language and communication disorders: I. Clinical assessment, definition of terms, and evaluation of their reliability. *Archives of General Psychiatry*, **36**, 1315–1321.
—— (1979b) Thought, language and communication disorders: II. Diagnostic significance. *Archives of General Psychiatry*, **36**, 1325–1330.
BERTELSON, P. (1986) The onset of literacy. *Cognition*, **24**, 1–30.
——, MORAIS, J., CARY, L., *et al* (1987) Interpreting data from illiterates: reply to Koopmans. *Cognition*, **27**, 113–115.

—— & DE GELDER, B. (1989) Learning about reading from illiterates. In *From Reading to Neurons* (ed. A. Galaburda), pp. 1–25. Cambridge, Mass.: MIT Press.
BLEULER, E. (1911) *Dementia Praecox or the Group of the Schizophrenias*. New York: International Universities Press (1966).
BOBON, J. (1947) Trois langues artificielles d'origine ludique chez un paraphrénique hypomaniaque. *Journal Belge de Neurologie*, **47**, 327–395.
BUCKINGHAM, H. W. & KERTESZ, A. (1976) *Neologistic Jargonaphasia*. Amsterdam: Swets & Zeitlinger.
CANCRO, R. (1983) History and overview of schizophrenia. In *Comprehensive Textbook of Psychiatry*, Vol. 1 (eds H. Kaplan & B. J. Sadock), pp. 631–643. Baltimore: Williams & Wilkins.
CÉNAC, M. (1925) *De Certains Langages Créés par les Aliénés: Contribution à l'Étude des Glossolalies*. Thèse de doctorat (Médecine), Université de Paris.
CHAIKA, E. O. (1974) A linguist looks at schizophrenic language. *Brain and Language*, **1**, 257–276.
FLOURNOY, Th. (1900) *Des Indes à la Planète Mars: Etude d'un Cas de Somnambulisme avec Glossolalie*. Paris: Alcan.
FREUD, S. (1910) The antithetical meaning of primal words. In *The Standard Edition of the Complete Psychological Works of Sigmund Freud, Volume XI* (ed. J. Strachey), pp. 155–161. London: Hogarth Press.
LECOURS, A. R. (1982a) On neologisms. In *Perspectives on Mental Representations* (eds J. Mehler, E. C. T. Walker & M. Garrett), pp. 217–250. Hillsdale, New Jersey: Lawrence Erlbaum.
—— (1982b) Simulation of speech production without a computer. In *Neural Models of Language Processes* (eds M. Arbib, J. Marshall & D. Caplan), pp. 345–367. New York: Academic Press.
—— & LHERMITTE, F. (1972) Recherches sur le langage des aphasiques: 4. Analyse d'un corpus de néologismes: notion de paraphasie monémique. *L'encéphale*, **61**, 295–315.
—— & VANIER-CLÉMENT, M. (1976) Schizophasia and jargonaphasia: a comparative description with comments on Chaika's and Fromkin's respective looks at schizophrenic language. *Brain and Language*, **3**, 516–565.
——, OSBORN, E., TRAVIS, L., *et al* (1981a) Jargons. In *Jargonaphasia* (ed. J. W. Brown), pp. 9–38. London: Academic Press.
——, NAVET, M. & ROSS, A. (1981b) Langage et pensée du schizophase. *Confrontations Psychiatriques*, **19**, 109–144.
LEVY-VALENSI, J., MIGAULT, P. & LACAN, J. (1931) Ecrits 'inspirés': schizographie. *Annales Médico-Psychologiques*, **89**, 1–26.
MANN, V. (1986) Phonological awareness: the role of reading experience. *Cognition*, **24**, 65–92.
MORAIS, J., CARY, L., ALEGRIA, J., *et al* (1979) Does awareness of speech as a sequence of phones arise spontaneously? *Cognition*, **7**, 323–331.
——, BERTELSON, P., CARY, L., *et al* (1986) Literacy training and speech segmentation. *Cognition*, **24**, 45–64.
POROT, A. (1975) *Manuel Alphabétique de Psychiatrie*. Paris: Presses Universitaires de France.
READ, CH, YUN-FEI, Z., HONG-YIN, N., *et al* (1986) The ability to manipulate speech sounds depends on knowing alphabetic writing. *Cognition*, **24**, 31–44.
SAMARIN, W. J. (1972) *Tongues of Men and Angels*. New York: MacMillan.
WEINER, H. (1983) Schizophrenia: etiology. In *Comprehensive Textbook of Psychiatry, Vol. 1* (eds H. Kaplan & B. J. Sadock), pp. 650–680. Baltimore: Williams & Wilkins.

8 Syntactic processing and communication disorder in first-onset schizophrenia

PHILIP THOMAS and IVAN LEUDAR

Some psychotic patients talk in a manner that listeners find extremely difficult to follow. Such patients are usually described as 'thought disordered' by clinicians, and the phenomenon has been widely regarded as diagnostic of schizophrenia (Edwards, 1972). The precise nature of the phenomenon remains obscure. Some (e.g. Lanin-Kettering & Harrow, 1985) maintain that the oddities of speech of such patients are part of a subset of abnormalities of behaviour including disordered thinking. Others (e.g. Chaika, 1982a) argue that the term 'thought disorder' is best replaced by 'speech disorder'. 'Schizophrenic thought disorder' would certainly appear to be problematic. It is difficult to measure reliably (Kreitman, 1962), may be tautological (Rochester & Martin, 1979), makes unwarranted assumptions about the relationship between thought and speech (Maher, 1972), and may be found in conditions other than schizophrenia (Andreasen, 1979a,b).

Recent developments in linguistics and cognitive science have considerably extended our understanding of thought disorder. There is evidence that the phenomenon is associated with disturbances in cohesion (Rochester & Martin, 1979; Harvey, 1983), an important feature of texts through which semantic relationships are established between sentences. Although the syntactic features of schizophrenic speech have been well characterised (Morice & Ingram, 1982; Fraser *et al*, 1986; Hoffman & Sledge, 1988), there have been no systematic studies of the syntactic aspect of the speech of patients with thought disorder. In any case, the exact significance of these linguistic studies is uncertain. Do they represent a distinct failure of linguistic competence? Or, as Schwartz (1982) suggests, are they merely secondary to the profound disturbances in cognition that occur in acute psychosis?

The act of communicating through speech is an extremely complex one. It involves higher cognitive processes such as the planning and monitoring of discourse, the successful direction of attention and working memory to subserve language, language processing itself, and social cognition (in essence, monitoring the needs, intentions and strategies of the listener).

One way of simplifying the situation is to examine linguistic performance in writing. Very little attention has been paid to written language in psychosis. Although linguistic skills in speaking and writing may be similar, the communicative intent in the two situations may be quite different. We speak to others with the intention of communicating in a social context. While we may write thus, such an act is usually free of the immediate social context – the person for whom the message is intended is not there. Linguistic studies of speech assess linguistic competence in the social act of communication. This depends upon the nature of the task studied, which should be naturalistic and representative of the use of language in its main function of social communication. Written language is interesting because it is not primarily an act of social communication. For this reason, it may be more sensitive to the effect of changes in language processing and cognitive factors relating to the illness.

There are difficulties here. How does one obtain written language? If subjects are asked to write an essay, several factors may influence performance, including motivation, interest and knowledge. It is almost impossible to standardise the difficulty of the task. One way of trying to do so was devised by Hunt (1970). The Hunt test consists of 32 input propositions in the form of simple sentences. Subjects are requested to rewrite these more concisely, including all the information from the original propositions. The subjects' responses are analysed to yield measures of syntactic maturity and complexity. Hunt (1970) followed the development of syntactic skills in normal school-age children. As they mature, children move from tensed verbal predicates and use adverbial and adjectival constructions, prepositional phrases and gerunds. Increasing linguistic ability is indicated by an increase both in clause length and syntactic complexity.

In view of the fact that the speech of schizophrenic people is syntactically distinct from that of other subjects, examining their written language on the Hunt test may help to elucidate the precise nature of the linguistic problem. The Hunt test minimises the role of social context and the subject's communicative intention. It may reflect the extent to which cognitive factors, in isolation, influence linguistic performance.

Hoffman *et al* (1985) studied the performance of schizophrenic and non-schizophrenic patients on the Hunt test. The schizophrenic subjects made more errors in representing the original input propositions, although there were no differences in complexity. Further analysis revealed that errors were particularly likely to occur when propositions were rewritten in the syntactically more complex passive voice. The authors claimed their results supported the existence of a failure of syntactic (language) processing in schizophrenia.

Thomas *et al* (1993) found that manic patients made similar errors, particularly while attempting syntactically more complex clause structures, suggesting that the problem is not specific to schizophrenia. As both schizophrenic and manic groups in that replication study contained subjects with severe communication disorder, the next task was to compare the performance of groups with and without communication disorder on the Hunt test. For this purpose we studied schizophrenic subjects only, for there were too few manic subjects to place in subgroups. We wanted to examine the extent to which problems in language processing on the Hunt test, if they existed, were accounted for by disturbances in cognition, particularly working memory and attention. The purpose of the study, therefore, was to investigate the following questions:

(a) Do communication-disordered schizophrenic subjects make more errors than schizophrenic subjects without communication disorder?
(b) Are these errors more likely to occur with more syntactically complex structures?
(c) Are errors accounted for by differences in cognition (working memory and attention) between the groups?

A study of written language in schizophrenia

Patients

Patients were recruited from acute admissions to two hospitals in Manchester, during a prospective study of negative symptoms in first-onset psychosis. Detailed selection and inclusion criteria for the patients in this study have been described by Montague *et al* (1989). For inclusion here, subjects had to be between 16 and 50 years old, within two years of the first appearance of psychotic symptoms, have no history of substance misuse, and have no evidence of organic brain syndromes or learning disability (i.e. completed normal schooling). All subjects had English as a first language. Clinical assessments were made within 72 hours of admission. Patients were assigned to diagnostic groups using the Research Diagnostic Criteria (RDC; Spitzer *et al*, 1975) derived from the Present State Examination (PSE; Wing *et al*, 1974).

There were 45 patients who met the RDC for definite or probable schizophrenia. They were placed in one of two groups, communication disordered (CD) and non-communication disordered (NCD) on the basis of the total score on the Thought Language and Communication Scale (TLC). This was used to measure frequency of communication abnormalities in the language interviews (see below). The median total score was 6, so the 15 subjects scoring more than this were categorised as CD. The 15 NCD subjects scored less than 2 on the TLC. The remaining 15 were excluded from the analysis.

Controls

Eighteen psychiatrically normal control subjects were recruited from acute admissions to an orthopaedic ward. These subjects were chosen to control for the non-specific effects of stress arising from sudden admission to hospital, and the possibility that these factors might influence language and communication. All controls were interviewed and screened with a structured questionnaire to exclude major psychiatric syndromes. No control subject suffered from psychiatric illness, or neurological disorders. Two were excluded because of a family history of psychiatric disorder, and three were excluded because of heavy alcohol intake.

Demographic characteristics

The demographic characteristics of the three groups of subjects (controls, CD schizophrenic and NCD schizophrenics) are compared in Table 8.1. There were no differences between the groups as far as medication (in chlorpromazine equivalents for the 72 hours before testing; Davis, 1974), and years of full-time education were concerned. Controls were, on average, a few years younger than both schizophrenic groups, although the difference is not statistically significant. They also achieved significantly higher academic standards, with an average attainment of A-levels, compared with the schizophrenic subjects' average of O-levels. There were no significant differences in the sex and social-class distributions of the two groups.

Assessments

The language interviews, lasting about 45 minutes, were undertaken by psychiatrically naïve psychology undergraduates, blind to diagnosis, within

TABLE 8.1
Demographic characteristics of subjects in study

	Mean	s.d.		
Age: years				
C	21.3	12.6		
NCD	26.4	5.2	$F = 2.01$	$P < 0.1$
CD	27.7	9.3		
Full-time education: years				
C	12.8	2.1		
NCD	13.0	2.6	$F = 1.10$	NS
CD	11.9	2.0		
Educational level[1]				
C	4.17	2.55		
NCD	3.80	1.97	$F = 3.94$	$P < 0.05$
CD	2.20	1.52		
Medication[2]				
NCD	1096	1792	$t = -1.26$, NS	
CD	1023	1345		

C = controls ($n = 18$); NCD = non-communication-disordered schizophrenic subjects ($n = 21$); CD = communication-disordered schizophrenic subjects ($n = 21$).
1. Coded as follows: 1 = none; 2 = CSEs; 3 = O-levels; 4 = A-levels; 5 = degree; 6 = postgraduate.
2. In mg, chlorpromazine equivalents.

the first week of admission. A proportion of patients were interviewed while on no medication. We performed correlations between neuroleptic medication at the time of testing and the Hunt test measures to see if any relationship existed. None of the correlations achieved statistical significance.

Subjects were given the Hunt test at the end of this interview, and were asked to complete it in their own time.

The Hunt test

The Hunt test consists of 32 single propositions in the form of simple sentences describing the manufacture of aluminium. It is an attempt to standardise the nature and difficulty of the task set to elicit written language output. It was originally devised to provide a simple and reliable method of assessing syntactic maturity in school children and adults. The analysis, details of which are presented in Appendix 1, produces measures of complexity and error. To analyse the subject's response to the test, it is necessary to identify lexical items, or their transformations, relating to each of the 32 input propositions. If no lexical item can be traced from an input proposition, that proposition is said to have been deleted in the subject's representation of the Hunt test material. In the next stage, the structural outcome for each input proposition is identified. There are five possible outcomes: main clause, coordinated predicate, subordinate clause, less than predicate, and proposition deletion (see Appendix 1 for examples). Sentence length, in words, is also measured.

Modifications to the Hunt test

Hoffman *et al* (1985) modified Hunt's analysis to produce error measures. This depends on whether the meaning of the input propositions can be extracted from the subject's text. For a successful representation, the text must not only convey the meaning of the original proposition, but it must do so in the sequence implied by the original proposition. In other words, it must be contextually correct. Hoffman describes three types of errors: syntactic, semantic, and contextual misrepresentations (see Appendix 1).

Hunt test measures

The Hunt test yields the following measures, all of which were used in the study:

(a) Complexity variables. Hunt's measures of written syntactic *maturity* are, strictly speaking, not the same as measures of *complexity* in studies of speech. This is because 'less than predicate' forms have no clausal structure, so they

cannot be said to measure syntactic complexity. Indeed, it is argued that the 'less than predicate' index is a measure of integration of information contained in the Hunt propositions, rather than syntactic complexity. Two other Hunt measures, the subordinate clause index and sentence length in words, are more clearly related to complexity measures. These scores were also used. Several of the Hunt test propositions are written in the active voice. The extent to which subjects rewrite these propositions in the passive voice is another important index of syntactic complexity. The voice of all sentences and clausal structures was identified, and classified as either active or passive, using criteria taken from a standard reference work of English grammar (Quirk *et al*, 1985). The mean number of passive clausal rewrites per subject was calculated.

(*b*) *Error variables*. The error score was calculated as the sum of the syntactically, semantically and contextually deviant representations. We repeated Hoffman's analysis to see if a relationship existed between syntactic complexity and error. Would subjects make more errors as they attempted to construct syntactically more complex outcomes? To investigate this, we noted the outcome for each Hunt sentence, paying particular attention to passive, less than predicate, and subordinate clause outcomes, the three most linguistically complex forms. The number of errors with each outcome was recorded. The number of errors occurring with a particular syntactic outcome through chance alone increases both as the number of errors increases and as the number of Hunt sentence deletions increases. As schizophrenic and manic subjects in the previous study deleted more sentences than controls, we used a mathematical model that took account of this. The hypergeometric distribution (Meyer, 1971) (Appendix 2) was therefore used to calculate a probability value for the association between error and complexity for each subject, accounting for the non-random nature of error occurrence. The mathematical details of this are given in Appendix 1. Interrater reliability for proposition outcome was satisfactory (weighted kappa = 0.88, $P < 0.05$), and for error scores (weighted kappa = 0.66, $0.05 > P > 0.1$).

(*c*) *Other measures of cognitive function*. Cognitive function is generally disturbed in acute psychoses. Without some measures of this disturbance, it is impossible to draw any conclusions as to the significance of any differences in language measures. Recent work suggests that working memory is particularly important as far as language is concerned. Baddeley (1986) has pointed out that it plays an important role in tasks such as holding the 'inner speech' needed for short-term memory tasks (e.g. remembering a name and address). Subjects have to store considerable amounts of information in short-term memory in the Hunt test. The successful completion of the test depends upon the successful location, storage and retrieval of information. Impairments in working memory are likely to have a significant influence on the Hunt test. Information will either be missed out (proposition deletion) or misrepresented (error outcome). We chose the reverse digit span test as a measure of working memory, and the shape cancelling test to provide a measure of subjects' attention.

(*i*) *Reverse digit span test.* In this test, the experimenter presents subjects with verbal sequences of digits, which they have to repeat backwards. In our test, we used a minimum sequence of two digits and a maximum of five. At each level the subject was asked to repeat backwards six sequences of digits. The total number of correct repetitions was taken as a score. The minimum was thus 0, the maximum 24.

(*ii*) *Shape cancelling test.* Here, subjects were presented with an A4 sheet with 891 randomly printed non-alphabetic and non-numeric characters – 33 columns and 27 rows of @ < > & % ! $? | *. Their task was to cancel all the right- or left-pointing arrows, of which there were 102. The numbers of correctly cancelled, omitted, and incorrectly cancelled characters were counted. Two indices were calculated: the relative frequency of characters incorrectly cancelled ('errors'); and the frequency of characters missed ('omissions'). These two measures are assumed to be measures of attention.

The point of these indices, of working memory (reverse digit span test) and attention (shape cancelling test), is to match the groups on some aspects of information processing. These measures reflect more directly the effect of severity of illness on cognition in psychosis.

Results

Between-group comparisons were made for controls, CD and NCD schizophrenic subjects, for each group of variables. The Kolmogorov–Smirnov goodness-of-fit test was used to establish whether the variables used approximated to a normal distribution. All variables meeting this criterion were examined either by analysis of variance with Scheffe's procedure to compare pairs of group means, or the t-test. Analysis of covariance was used to compare group effects and the interaction with covariates. There were differences in the sizes of the three groups, and, for some variables, the homogeneity of the variance. These were analysed non-parametrically using the Mann–Whitney test to compare pairs of groups, or the Kruskall–Wallis one-way analysis of variance for the three groups. All data were analysed using the Statistical Package for the Social Sciences (Nie *et al*, 1975).

Complexity

The results of the Hunt test are presented in Table 8.2. In general there are few differences between the three groups. The exception is the 'less than predicate' score, where control subjects, on average, produced two and a half times as many 'less than predicate' outcomes than CD schizophrenic subjects, with NCD schizophrenic subjects falling between the two. This

TABLE 8.2
Complexity scores from the Hunt test

	Mean score	s.d.		
Mean clause length: words				
C	7.5	1.2		
NCD	7.3	3.6	$F = 1.36$,	NS
CD	6.2	1.3		
Mean sentence length: words				
C	14.6	4.0		
NCD	15.5	8.9	$F = 0.12$,	NS
CD	16.0	11.2		
Subordinate clause index				
C	4.17	2.12		
NCD	3.07	2.34	$F = 0.82$,	NS
CD	3.47	3.04		
Less than predicate score				
C[1]	13.8	5.6		
NCD	8.7	5.8	$F = 10.99$,	$P < 0.01$
CD[1]	5.3	4.2		
Mean passive outcomes				
C	3.17	2.63		
NCD	2.27	2.79	$F = 2.89$,	$0.1 > P > 0.05$
CD	1.40	1.60		

1. C significantly >CD, using Scheffe's test.
For key to abbreviations see Table 8.1.

indicates that controls are able to integrate the information from the input propositions more successfully. Controls tend to use more passive outcomes than the patient groups, although this difference is not significant at the 5% level.

We found significant correlations between educational attainment and the 'less than predicate' score ($r = 0.50$), so we performed an analysis of covariance to examine the effects of these two variables and group membership. A significant effect was found for educational attainment ($F = 24.01$, $P < 0.01$), but a significant group effect remained ($F = 7.13$, $P < 0.05$). This indicates that the group differences in the 'less than predicate' score were not simply explained by the differences in educational attainment.

Error

The results of the error analysis (Table 8.3) reveal marked differences between the three groups. CD subjects produce more semantically and syntactically (ungrammatical) anomalous propositions and make more contextually anomalous propositions. Overall, the CD group make on average five times as many errors as controls, and three times as many as the NCD group, as shown by the total error score. There was, however, a significant negative correlation between total error score and educational

TABLE 8.3
Error scores from the Hunt test

	Mean	s.d.
Semantically anomalous		
C	20.1	
NCD	21.2	$\chi^2 = 8.00$, $P<0.05$
CD	33.1	
Contextually anomalous		
C	20.7	
NCD	22.7	$\chi^2 = 5.62$, $P<0.05$
CD	30.8	
Ungrammatical outcomes		
C	21.3	
NCD	21.8	$\chi^2 = 6.50$, $P<0.05$
CD	31.1	
Total error score		
C	0.72	1.48
NCD	1.27	2.34, $F = 8.03$, $P<0.01$
CD	4.80	3.69

χ^2 calculated using Kruskal–Wallis one-way analysis of variance.
F calculated using one-way analysis of variance.
For key to abbreviations see Table 8.1.

attainment ($r = -0.40$), so analysis of covariance was performed to examine the interaction of error, educational attainment, and group membership. A significant effect was found for educational attainment ($F = 14.93$, $P<0.01$), although a significant group effect remained ($F = 7.02$, $P<0.01$), suggesting that the high error rate of the CD group was not simply explained by their lower educational attainment.

Do subjects make more errors as they attempt syntactically more complex forms? To investigate this, the probability of associations between error and outcome were rank ordered and the mean rank for each group compared using the Mann–Whitney test, corrected for ties. It was predicted that CD schizophrenic subjects would make significantly more errors than NCD schizophrenic subjects while attempting more complex structures. The controls were excluded from this part of the analysis because of their low error rate. Both 'subordinate clauses' and 'less than predicate' outcomes were significantly more likely to be associated with errors, according to this analysis. For CD schizophrenic subjects the mean ranks for these two variables were 18.60 and 17.40 ($Z = -1.66$ and -2.27 respectively), compared with 23.29 and 24.43 for NCD schizophrenic subjects. There was no difference between the two groups as far as errors with passive outcomes were concerned.

Measures of cognition

The results of the tests of working memory (reverse digit span) and attention (shape cancelling test) are found in Table 8.4. The performance of control

TABLE 8.4
Results for working memory and attention

	Mean	s.d.		
Working memory				
C	0.84	0.16		
NCD	0.66	0.26	$F = 5.97$,	$P < 0.01$
CD	0.56	0.24		
Shape cancelling test: errors				
C	0.02	0.02		
NCD	0.07	0.10	$F = 2.58$,	$0.05 < P < 0.1$
CD	0.10	0.12		
Shape cancelling test: omissions				
C	0.08	0.08		
NCD	0.23	0.36	$F = 2.60$,	$0.05 < P < 0.1$
CD	0.29	0.30		

For key to abbreviations see Table 8.1.

subjects on the reverse digit span test was significantly better than that of CD schizophrenic subjects (Scheffe's test), and they also tended to do better on the shape cancelling test (errors and omissions scores) than either patient groups, although the results here just fail to reach significance at the 5% level.

We found significant correlations between 'less than predicate' score, working memory ($r = 0.36$) and attention (errors, $r = -0.40$; omissions, $r = -0.38$), as well as Hunt test total error score with working memory ($r = -0.46$) and attention (errors, $r = 0.49$; omissions, $r = 0.40$). In view of this, the working-memory and attention variables were used as covariates in the analysis of the Hunt test scores. For 'less than predicate' score, both working memory ($F = 5.51$, $P < 0.05$) and attention (errors, $F = 6.20$, $P < 0.05$) had significant effects, but significant group differences remained ($F = 3.81$, $P < 0.05$). Similarly, for the Hunt test total error score, both working memory ($F = 11.19$, $P < 0.01$) and attention (errors, $F = 13.89$, $P < 0.01$) had significant effects, but significant group differences remained ($F = 4.03$, $P < 0.05$). These results suggest that the group differences in working memory and attention account for some of the differences in language processing, as measured by the 'less than predicate' and Hunt test error scores, but there are still significant group differences.

Discussion

There are no differences between control subjects and the two groups of schizophrenic subjects for most of the Hunt test measures except 'less than predicate' outcomes, which CD schizophrenic subjects use less frequently. Hunt claimed that this measure is a particularly sensitive index of syntactic maturity. Although our subjects' performance was partially explained by educational attainment, this did not explain all the variance on this measure. Significant group differences remained. While it may be a sensitive measure of syntactic maturity, the 'less than predicate' score probably reflects a higher-order cognitive process involved in the integration of information. In order to produce such outputs in the Hunt test, it is necessary to hold large amounts of information in working memory. We found that both working memory and attention significantly influenced 'less than predicate' score, indicating the importance of these aspects of cognitive function in language processing. However, not all the variance in this score was explained by these measures of cognition. Significant group differences persisted. This indicates that the poor performance of the CD schizophrenic subjects was not simply explained by their impaired cognitive function. It suggests that they have an independent deficit in language processing.

The CD schizophrenic subjects consistently made more errors than the other groups, but there were no differences in the error scores of control and NCD schizophrenic subjects. This is important. It is the first time that subjects who have communication disorder in speech have been shown to have problems in language processing in written tasks. Although educational attainment explained a significant amount of the variance in error score, the group differences remained. Both working memory and attention had a significant influence on the error score, but again, significant group differences remained. Although non-specific disruption of cognitive processes has an important influence on linguistic performance as measured by the Hunt test error score, it does not provide a complete picture. Communication disorder in acute psychosis would appear to be associated with a specific language-processing disorder on the basis of these results. This is further supported by the association between error and complexity of outcome. CD schizophrenic subjects were more likely to make errors while generating syntactically more complex 'subordinate clause' and 'less than predicate' structures. This indicates that, as they tried to use more complex syntactic forms, they made more errors. This can be taken as further evidence that CD schizophrenic subjects have a specific defect in linguistic processing quite unrelated to the effects of cognition.

To what extent do these findings elucidate the likely nature of the linguistic failure in communication disorder in schizophrenia? Garrett (1975) has developed a complex model of sentence production based on a detailed analysis of thousands of speech errors made by healthy subjects. He proposes that communicative intention is translated into a set of instructions which guide the articulatory apparatus. These instructions require distinct levels of syntactic analysis (processing), one of which determines the grammatical relationship of words and phrases, while another is responsible for the serial ordering of 'content' words. Although the initial stage (formation of a communicative intention) and final stage (writing, not speaking) of the Hunt test are quite different, there is no reason to suppose that the intermediate stages of syntactic processing differ from those of speech. To what extent are the results in this study explicable in terms of a disruption of these intermediate stages of Garrett's model?

Hoffman & Sledge (1984) have argued that the main difference between 'normal' and 'schizophrenic' speakers is that normal subjects make errors within an intact syntactic framework (that is, the first level described above), which, in schizophrenic speakers, is disrupted. The Hunt test errors include syntactic, semantic and contextual varieties. The last may be viewed as a disruption of the propositional equivalent of the second stage of Garrett's model, whereby, instead of the serial ordering of 'content' words being disrupted, the serial ordering of the Hunt test propositions is disrupted. That CD schizophrenic subjects make significantly more syntactically deviant (ungrammatical) constructions supports Hoffman's interpretation of Garrett's theory, that CD schizophrenic subjects have a deviant syntactic framework. The input propositions are not in themselves syntactically deviant, but in rewriting them, subjects are increasing the complexity of the clausal structure. As they do so, they make more errors. This is confirmed by the observation that errors are more likely to be associated with increasingly complex structures. It suggests that the constraints exerted by the syntactic framework of the CD subjects induce errors, as they attempt to convey the complex relationships between Hunt propositions in a more concise form. However, NCD schizophrenic subjects also tend to make more contextual errors, which suggests that there is, in addition, a disturbance at the level of proposition organisation. This is consistent with the evidence that the speech of schizophrenic subjects is poorly linked above the sentence level, because of problems in the use of cohesive ties.

This explanation is more systematic than that propounded by Chaika (1982b) which attempts to relate deviant schizophrenic utterance to random triggering of words and inappropriate perseveration. Such a model cannot explain the relationship between syntactic complexity and errors. The Hoffman/Garrett model is more satisfactory from this point of view, because the more complex the sentence, the greater the likelihood that the serial ordering will be confused, or the grammatical structure will suffer, or information will be missed out. This is confirmed by the observation that CD schizophrenic subjects make more omissions than the other two groups.

A note of caution is necessary, however. Another study of the same subjects (Thomas *et al*, 1993) found that manic patients had virtually the same pattern of performance on the Hunt test as schizophrenic patients. Although manic subjects were not included in this study, the most parsimonious conclusion would be that the performance of manic subjects with CD would be similar to that of CD schizophrenic subjects on the Hunt test. In other words, this study's findings relate only to the phenomenon of communication disorder, and are of little importance as far as different diagnostic groups are concerned. This supports Bentall's view (1990) that future research should concentrate on the relationship between specific symptoms, such as communication disorder or verbal hallucinations, and cognitive abnormalities, rather than diagnostic entities which are probably too broad and heterogeneous to yield useful results.

Acknowledgements

Dr Thomas, who was in receipt of a Wellcome travel grant at the time, is grateful to Professor Ralph Hoffman, University of Yale Department of Psychiatry, for his time and help in advising on the Hunt test analysis.

Appendix 1. The Hunt test

The propositions are as follows:

> Aluminium is a metal (P1). It is abundant (P2). It has many uses (P3). It comes from bauxite (P4). Bauxite is an ore (P5). Bauxite looks like clay (P6). Bauxite contains aluminium (P7). It contains several other substances (P8). Workmen extract these other substances from the bauxite (P9). They grind the bauxite (P10). They put it in tanks (P11). Pressure is in the tanks (P12). The other substances form a mass (P13). They remove the mass (P14). They use filters (P15). A liquid remains (P16). They put it through several other processes (P17). It finally yields a chemical (P18). The chemical is powdery (P19). It is white (P20). The chemical is alumina (P21). It is a mixture (P22). It contains aluminium (P23). It contains oxygen (P24). Workmen separate the aluminium from the oxygen (P25). They use electricity (P26). They finally produce a metal (P27). The metal is light (P28). It has a lustre (P29). The lustre is bright (P30). The lustre is silvery (P31). This metal comes in many forms (P32).

The following example of the Hunt test was produced by the project linguist (MJ), who has an honours degree in English, and who has not studied chemistry:

> Aluminium, an abundant metal with many uses, is obtained by grinding a clay-like ore called bauxite and putting it in pressurised tanks, so that the liquid which can then be filtered off from the coagulated impurities will, after several other processes, yield the powdery white chemical alumina, which, when the oxygen has been removed electrically, finally produces a light metal with a bright silvery lustre, available in many forms.

The Hunt test was analysed in four ways to produce measures of complexity, error and voice (passive/active).

Complexity

To analyse the test it is necessary to identify the outcome, in the completed text, of each sentence in the original paragraph. There are five possible outcomes:

(a) *Main clause* – the subject and predicate of the original sentence remain as a main clause.
Example   Bauxite is a clay-like ore.

Proposition 5 in the Hunt test ("Bauxite is an ore") is represented as a main clause, with proposition 6 ("Bauxite looks like clay") reduced to the composite adjective "clay-like". This lacks clausal structure and is thus a 'less than predicate' outcome for proposition 6 (see (d), below)

(b) *Coordinated predicate* – the subject of the original preposition is left out, but the predicate remains tensed and coordinated to another main clause.
Example   It comes in many forms and has many uses.

Proposition 3 is here expressed as a coordinated predicate, sharing the same subject, "It" (referring to this metal, or aluminium), as proposition 32, which is represented as a main clause.

(c) *Subordinate clause* – the subject and predicate of the original sentence remain as the subject and tensed predicate of a subordinate clause, under a main clause.
Example   which contains aluminium and other substances.

Proposition 7 is expressed as a subordinate clause and proposition 8 is reduced to a 'less than predicate' outcome.

(d) *Less than predicate* – this includes any non-clausal outcome for the original proposition (nouns, adjectives, adverbs, gerunds, etc.) – see example in (a).

(e) *Sentence deletion* – no information from the original sentence is present in the completed text.

With the exception of sentence deletions, all the above measures were used by Hunt. The validity of two measures, the 'less than predicate' index (the total number of 'less than predicate' outcomes for each subject) and clause length (the total number of words divided by the total number of main and subordinate clauses), is very high when judged against school grade. It will be clear that the more 'less than predicate' forms a subject uses, the less likely he/she will be to use tensed clausal structures and embedding.

Error measures

(a) *Syntactically deviant* – the information from the original sentence is contained in a structure that is ungrammatical.
Example   The ( ) is bright.

The lexical items in the rewrite are derived from proposition 30, but the sentence lacks a subject and is thus syntactically deviant.

(b) *Semantically deviant* – although information from the original is present, the meaning of the original is not successfully represented.
Example   The lustre is silvery and metallic and is produced in many forms.

Proposition 32 states that the metal (aluminium) comes in many forms. This patient has substituted the noun 'lustre' from proposition 29 as the subject of a coordinated predicate, with the result that the meaning of proposition 32 is lost. It is therefore semantically deviant.

(c) *Contextually deviant* – although information from the original is present, its meaning is lost because it occurs out of sequence with adjacent sentences.
Example Workmen extract their substances from the pressure ( ) is in the tank

In this example proposition 12 occurs out of context, so proposition 12 is contextually deviant. It is also syntactically deviant because it should presumably form a subordinate clause, but the subordinator 'which' is missing.

Voice (passive/active)

Example After being in the pressure tank a mass is formed.

Proposition 13, which occurs in the active voice in its original form, is rewritten in the passive voice.

Appendix 2. The hypergeometric distribution

Let T elements be divided into K classes in a given sample. Let $T_1\ T_2\ \ldots\ T_k$ be the number of elements in the K classes. Then

$$T_i = T$$

A random sample of N elements with replacement contains n_1 of class 1, n_2 of class 2 . . . n_k of class k, so that $n_i = N$

The probability of occurrence of such a sample according to the hypergeometric distribution is:

$$\frac{\begin{array}{cccc}T_1 & T_2 & \ldots & T_k \\ n_1 & n_2 & \ldots & n_k\end{array}}{\begin{array}{c}T \\ N\end{array}}$$

This method can be used as described by Hoffman to estimate the non-randomness of errors occurring with passive forms, subordinate clauses, and less than predicate outcomes, using the following formula:

$$Pr(e=i) = \frac{\begin{array}{cc}p & 32-D-p \\ i & e-i\end{array}}{\begin{array}{c}32-D \\ e\end{array}} = P(p, D, e, i)$$

Where: 32 = the total number of Hunt sentences
   D = the total number of deletions
   $(32 - D) = T$; the total sample space
   p = total number of passive rewrites
   $(32 - D - p)$ = total number of non-passive rewrites
   e = total number of errors
   i = total number of errors in passive rewrites
   $(e - i)$ = errors occurring with non-passive rewrites

For errors occurring with less than predicate and subordinated clauses, the values of p and i change accordingly.

References

ANDREASEN, N. C. (1979a) Thought, language and communication disorders: I. Clinical assessment, definition of terms, and evaluation of their reliability. *Archives of General Psychiatry*, **36**, 1315–1321.
—— (1979b) Thought, language and communication disorders: II. Diagnostic significance. *Archives of General Psychiatry*, **36**, 1325–1330.
BADDELEY, A. (1986) *Working Memory*. Oxford: Oxford University Press.
BENTALL, R. P. (ed.) (1990) *Reconstructing Schizophrenia*. London: Methuen.
CHAIKA, E. (1982a) Thought disorder or speech disorder in schizophrenia? *Schizophrenia Bulletin*, **8**, 587–591.
—— (1982b) A unified explanation for the diverse structural deviations reported for adult schizophrenics with disrupted speech. *Journal of Communication Disorders*, **15**, 167–189.
DAVIS, J. M. (1974) Dose equivalence of the antipsychotic drugs. *Journal of Psychiatric Research*, **11**, 65–69.
EDWARDS, G. (1972) Diagnosis of schizophrenia: an Anglo-American comparison. *British Journal of Psychiatry*, **120**, 385–390.
FRASER, W. I., KING, K., THOMAS, P., *et al* (1986) The diagnosis of schizophrenia by language analysis. *British Journal of Psychiatry*, **148**, 275–278.
GARRETT, M. (1975) The analysis of sentence production. In *The Psychology of Learning and Motivation* (ed. G. Bower), pp. 133–177. New York: Academic Press.
HARVEY, P. D. (1983) Speech competence in manic and schizophrenic psychosis: the association between clinically rated thought disorder and cohesion and reference performance. *Journal of Abnormal Psychology*, **92**, 368–377.
HOFFMAN, R. & SLEDGE, W. (1984) A microgenetic model of paragrammatisms produced by a schizophrenic speaker. *Brain and Language*, **21**, 147–173.
——, HOGBEN, G. L., SMITH, H., *et al* (1985) Message disruption during syntactic processing in schizophrenia. *Journal of Communication Disorders*, **18**, 183–202.
—— & SLEDGE, W. (1988) An analysis of grammatical deviance occurring in spontaneous schizophrenic speech. *Journal of Neurolinguistics*, **3**, 89–191.
HUNT, K. W. (1970) Syntactic maturity in school children and adults. *Monographs in Social Research and Child Development*, **35**, 1–67.
KREITMAN, N. (1962) The reliability of psychiatric assessment: an analysis. *Journal of Mental Science*, **107**, 887–908.
LANIN-KETTERING, I. & HARROW, M. (1985) The thought behind the words: a view of schizophrenic speech and thinking disorders. *Schizophrenia Bulletin*, **11**, 1–7.
MAHER, B. (1972) The language of schizophrenia: a review and interpretation. *British Journal of Psychiatry*, **120**, 3–17.
MEYER, P. L. (1971) *Introductory Probability and Statistical Applications*. Addison-Wesley.

MONTAGUE, L. R., TANTAM, D., NEWBY, D., et al (1989) The incidence of negative symptoms in early schizophrenia, mania and other psychoses. *Acta Psychiatrica Scandinavica*, **79**, 613–618.

MORICE, R. D. & INGRAM, J. C. L. (1982) Language analysis in schizophrenia: diagnostic implications. *Australian and New Zealand Journal of Psychiatry*, **16**, 11–21.

NIE, N. H., HULL, C. H., JENKINS, J., et al (1975) *Statistical Package for the Social Sciences*. New York: McGraw Hill.

QUIRK, R., GREENBAUM, S., LEECH, G., et al (1985) *A Comprehensive Grammar of the English Language*. London: Longman.

ROCHESTER, S. R. & MARTIN, J. R. (1979) *Crazy Talk: A Study of the Discourse of Schizophrenic Speakers*. New York: Plenum Press.

SCHWARTZ, S. (1982) Is there a schizophrenic language? *Behavioural and Brain Sciences*, **5**, 579–626.

SPITZER, R., ENDICOTT, J. & ROBINS, E. (1975) *Research Diagnostic Criteria. Instrument Number 58*. New York: New York State Psychiatric Institute.

THOMAS, P., LEUDAR, I., NEWBY, D., et al (1993) Syntactic processing and written language output in first onset psychosis. *Journal of Communication Disorders*, **26**, 209–230.

WING, J. K., COOPER, J. E. & SARTORIUS, N. (1974) *Measurement and Classification of Psychiatric Syndromes: An Instruction Manual for the PSE and CATEGO Programme*. Cambridge: Cambridge University Press.

9 The psychology of schizophrenic thought; the neuropsychology of schizophrenic speech

PETER McKENNA

As one of the few 'signs' in schizophrenia – that is, an objectively evident abnormality as opposed to one whose existence has to be inferred from subjective reports – it might be anticipated that formal thought disorder would be particularly susceptible to experimental investigation. Unfortunately, despite years of research, it is fair to say that what makes the speech of some schizophrenic patients difficult to follow remains an almost complete mystery.

At a phenomenological level, considerable progress has certainly been made in describing and classifying formal thought disorder. As a result of the work of numerous authors (see Andreasen, 1979; Sims, 1988), it is now accepted that thought-disordered schizophrenic speech is made up of several distinct abnormalities which may occur in any combination in any particular patient. These abnormalities span a number of levels: from disturbances in the organisation of thematic narratives (e.g. poverty of content of speech, loss of goal); through loosening of the associations between concepts (e.g. derailment, tangentiality); to disorders which might be referred to as quasi-linguistic, where the mechanisms governing word choice and sentence construction seem to be at fault (e.g. neologisms, word approximations, agrammatism).

The research which has attempted to explain what underlies and gives rise to the phenomena of formal thought disorder forms a voluminous literature which is larger than that on the rest of schizophrenic psychopathology put together. The task of attempting to review this literature can be simplified somewhat by distinguishing two broad approaches within it: the psychological and the neuropsychological. The former attempts to understand formal thought disorder as a disturbance in one or more normal cognitive functions. The latter merely screens patients with schizophrenia for evidence of disorders of language similar to those seen in neurological disease.

Evaluation of the psychological and neuropsychological findings can be simplified further still by considering them in the light of two fundamental methodological requirements. One of these is an axiom of psychological research in schizophrenia, that any abnormality found should not merely be part of the general tendency to poor performance which characterises the disorder. As emphasised by Chapman & Chapman (1973), patients with schizophrenia are notorious for performing poorly on virtually any psychological test that is set them, and so a performance decrement on a particular task does not necessarily mean that there is a specific impairment in that domain of cognitive function. A similar (or the same) principle applies to neuropsychological studies, as the well established finding that schizophrenia is associated with overall intellectual deterioration. This may range from a decline in IQ (e.g. Payne, 1973) to, in a minority of patients with the most severe and chronic forms of illness, something that amounts to what is to all intents and purposes a dementia (e.g. Owens & Johnstone, 1980; Liddle & Crow, 1984). In these circumstances, once again, poor performance on a specific test does not necessarily imply a specific neuropsychological deficit.

To avoid this pitfall in psychological studies without being so stringent as to exclude every study, a reasonable stipulation might be that any alleged abnormality should be demonstrable in acute schizophrenic patients, in whom the general tendency to poor performance is widely accepted as being least marked. In the case of neuropsychological studies, some measure should be included to show that the deficit found is disproportionate to any accompanying overall intellectual impairment.

The other requirement is that any psychological or neuropsychological abnormality which is claimed to be relevant to formal thought disorder should be associated with the presence of formal thought disorder clinically – that is, it should be present only in thought-disordered patients, or be at least most pronounced in these. Although this point might seem self-evident, it is surprising how often it has been ignored. As far as psychological studies are concerned, its neglect has had serious consequences in one well-known area of research (see below). With respect to neuropsychological studies, it is possible that a more explicit acknowledgement may help clarify the longstanding controversy about the relationship of formal thought disorder to dysphasia.

The psychology of formal thought disorder

Empirically oriented approaches

The emergence of the scientific discipline of psycholinguistics in the 1950s played a pivotal historical role in the approach taken to the study of thought disorder in schizophrenia. Inspired by the work of Chomsky and also by the development of several practical measures for assessing speech in an objective, quantitative way, psychologists set about analysing the verbal output of patients with schizophrenia. Typically, speech samples from schizophrenic patients were surveyed to determine if quantitative differences from normal speech could be demonstrated. Approaches taken included analysis of information content and redundancy (the best-known technique in this area being the cloze procedure), and examination of whether certain statistical regularities found in normal speech are also present in schizophrenia (e.g. the proportion of subjects to objects, and the type : token ratio between total words and different words used).

The findings of these studies have been reviewed many times (Maher, 1972; Schwartz, 1982; Rochester & Martin, 1979; Cutting, 1985). To summarise briefly, it is quite well established that schizophrenic speech contains less redundancy than normal speech, is less predictable, and contains less information. It is less clear whether schizophrenic patients use more subjects than objects, or have a type : token ratio that is different from normal. Schizophrenic patients show a slight tendency to repetitiveness. Some evidence has also suggested that they have a more restricted vocabulary than normal people.

As Maher (1972) put it, these findings provide a somewhat limited basis for the understanding of psychotic utterances, and it is only the first of them which appears to be at all relevant to the question of what makes schizophrenic speech difficult to follow. A more important failing of the studies in this area is that many of them did not meet the first of the requirements stated above, that the abnormality in question be demonstrable in acute schizophrenic patients, where the confounding effects of general tendency to poor performance are least evident. Findings like less information content and restriction of vocabulary can be plausibly construed as the consequences of a general intellectual decline on language function. A surprisingly large proportion of these studies have also failed to meet the second requirement, of specifying that the patient samples are restricted to those showing formal thought disorder.

Theoretically oriented approaches

Studies of this type have taken the classic experimental psychological approach of postulating a cognitive disorder to account for formal thought disorder, and then proceeding to test whether or not this can be demonstrated in thought-disordered patients. Somewhat surprisingly, only two main avenues have been explored in this way. One of these has been Rochester & Martin's (1979) hypothesis of an abnormality at the level of discourse, and the other has been Cameron's (1939, 1944) concept of overinclusive thinking.

Rochester & Martin took as their starting point one aspect of language use which they suspected might be particularly relevant to formal thought disorder – the way in which statements are linked together by the speaker into connected 'texts' of discourse. Just as the writer of a review article tries to maximise the intelligibility of the topic by ordering the findings in a logical way and continually reminding readers of this with headings and subheadings, speakers engaged in everyday conversations also abide by various rules and employ a variety of linguistic devices ('cohesive ties') in order to ensure that their message will get across clearly. Stripped of these, speech would merely be a jumble of not very well formed ideas, perhaps resembling the above writer's first draft. If schizophrenic patients failed to follow these rules, their speech might well come to be designated as abnormal in form, or in other words showing formal thought disorder.

Rochester & Martin went on to analyse the verbal output of two groups of acute schizophrenic patients. One of these was rated clinically as showing formal thought disorder and the other showed no evidence of this. A control group of normal subjects was also tested. Transcripts of the speech of all three groups were analysed for the presence of various classes of cohesive tie. It was found that the thought-disordered but not the non-thought-disordered schizophrenic patients used significantly fewer such ties; in particular, there was a lack of ties referring the listener to context. The contribution made by this abnormality to the clinical impression of formal thought disorder was substantial, but it was clear that it did not provide a complete explanation of the phenomenon.

A recent replication of Rochester & Martin's study (Chaika & Lambe, 1989; see also Chapter 4) had less impressive findings. Acute schizophrenic patients with formal thought disorder differed significantly from normals in only one out of six categories of cohesive tie measured.

Cameron's (1939, 1944) proposal of overinclusive thinking refers to an inability to select, eliminate and restrict thought to the task in hand, causing concepts to lose their sharp boundaries and closely or even distantly related ideas to merge into one another. As well as resulting in the expression of ideas which would appear vague and whimsical, overinclusiveness could cause the mental set of the speaker to cease to correspond to that of the listener, so that the train of thought would become difficult to follow. The same abnormality might also affect the choice of words and phrases, and so give rise to quasi-linguistic abnormalities.

The experimental investigation of overinclusive thinking was undertaken not by Cameron, but principally by Payne and co-workers (see Payne, 1973). Using procedures such as requiring subjects to give synonyms for words and sort pictures into conceptual categories, these authors repeatedly found that schizophrenic patients were significantly more overinclusive than normal individuals or non-psychotic patients. In several cases the findings were replicated in independent studies.

Later, in response to methodological criticisms and a number of reports of overinclusiveness in other patient groups, Payne and colleagues carried out a further series of studies using a battery of tests of overinclusiveness whose validity could be independently demonstrated. The results of these

TABLE 9.1
Combined overinclusiveness scores in various diagnostic groups (from Payne, 1973)

Diagnosis	Mean	s.d.	Number of cases
Paranoid schizophrenia	8.7	3.7	38
Non-paranoid schizophrenia	9.0	4.1	55
Acute schizophrenia	10.0	4.5	20
Chronic schizophrenia	5.3	2.4	17
Mania	10.9	4.6	13
Depression	6.3	3.0	41
Organic syndrome	11.6	3.5	7
Alcoholism	8.0	2.9	12
Personality disorder	7.1	2.9	20
Neurosis	7.3	2.9	55
Normals	4.9	1.6	20

'second-generation' studies are shown in Table 9.1. Almost no normal or neurotic patients obtained a combined overinclusiveness score comparable to that of the schizophrenic group as a whole. High overinclusiveness scores, however, were not exclusive to schizophrenia, also being found in mania and a small group of patients with organic disorders.

Overinclusive thinking amply fulfils the requirement of being present in acute schizophrenic patients. It is apparent from Table 9.1 that the phenomenon is in fact more characteristic of acute schizophrenia than chronic schizophrenia – chronic patients were no more overinclusive than neurotic patients, whereas the acute schizophrenic group contained a sizable proportion with the highest scores of any group. This finding has also been independently replicated (Harrow & Quinlan, 1985).

Does overinclusive thinking surmount the final hurdle of being associated with formal thought disorder? The available evidence suggests that unfortunately this is not the case. Hawks & Payne (1971) correlated performance on their combined overinclusiveness battery with clinicians' ratings of symptoms in 54 schizophrenic patients. It was found that overinclusiveness was significantly associated with a number of symptoms which are more or less typical of acute, florid schizophrenia: hostility, a high level of motor activity, talkativeness, and increased verbal responsiveness. There was no consistent relationship to presence of delusions. With respect to clinically evident formal thought disorder, however, the correlation was significantly inverse.

Summary

The experimental psychological investigation of formal thought disorder has not had any outstanding successes. Only overinclusive thinking stands out as a robust finding, having been demonstrated in a variety of test procedures and also having been independently replicated on a number of occasions. In addition, as pointed out by Chapman & Chapman (1973), it is the only psychological abnormality which has ever been found to be more characteristic of acute schizophrenia than chronic schizophrenia. Nevertheless, what evidence there is points squarely to the conclusion that overinclusiveness is not at all closely related to the clinical phenomenon it was originally invoked to explain.

The neuropsychology of schizophrenic speech

Studies of unselected schizophrenic patients

As with the empirically oriented cognitive psychological approach described above, a popular neuropsychological strategy has been to screen unselected groups of schizophrenic patients for evidence of impairments – phonemic, syntactic, or semantic. Many of the studies in this area have been reviewed by Cutting (1985).

With respect to phonemics, Cutting (1985) concluded that, notwithstanding scattered reports that schizophrenic patients misperceived words, it was doubtful whether there was evidence of any marked abnormalities of this type in their speech. There appears to have been no further work in this area.

Concerning syntactic abnormalities, Cutting (1985) found no evidence of changes in the use of words of different grammatical classes (i.e. nouns, verbs, adjectives) in schizophrenia. Some initial studies reporting that schizophrenic patients failed to appreciate syntactic complexity were subsequently not replicated. Various studies examining the understanding of sentences with increasingly complex grammar also found no real evidence of impairment.

These studies on the receptive aspects of syntax have been complemented by a series of studies which have examined the syntactic structure of schizophrenic patients' expressed speech. Analysing transcripts of free speech, Morice & Ingram (1982) and Fraser et al (1986) found that schizophrenic patients made significantly more syntactic errors than normal subjects, and that their speech was characterised by decreased syntactic complexity. However, these studies did not include any measure of overall intellectual impairment, and this may have been an important determinant of the findings. Thus, a later study by Fraser's group (Thomas et al, 1990) found that chronic schizophrenic patients showed more impairment on almost all of the measures of syntactic performance than acute patients, who were in turn worse than normal individuals. As Thomas et al (1990) pointed out, one explanation for this finding is simply that it reflected an overall deterioration in cognitive performance as the disorder progressed.

Cutting (1985) reviewed a number of studies of semantic language function in schizophrenia. Based on a variety of mainly receptive tests, for example, the ability to extract meaning (the 'gist') from sentences, he concluded that the semantic component of language was not obviously deranged in the large majority of patients with schizophrenia. A somewhat smaller number of studies has examined the semantic content of schizophrenic patients' expressed speech. These have been reviewed by Frith & Allen (1988), who concluded that the findings were contradictory, with some authors finding decreased meaningfulness and semantic deviance whereas others failed to replicate this. Once again, none of these studies controlled for overall intellectual impairment, and when impairment was found it tended to be maximal in chronic schizophrenic patients.

These studies present a mixed picture. The degree of abnormality – semantic or syntactic, receptive or expressive – is slight, and sometimes fails to show up at all. Where impairment is found, it seems to be associated with chronic illness. Few if any of these studies took the precaution of controlling for overall intellectual impairment, and so perhaps the simplest interpretation is that basic linguistic competence is compromised in schizophrenia only to a degree consistent with any accompanying general intellectual impairment.

These studies invariably also failed to restrict their patient samples to those with formal thought disorder, and it is therefore not clear that any abnormalities found have anything to do with formal thought disorder. This shortcoming, in contrast, leaves open the possibility that significant abnormality might be present in thought-disordered patients, but that this is swamped by normal performance in the large majority without this symptom. There is some reason to suspect that this might be the case: in a study of semantic abnormalities in schizophrenic speech, Cutting (1985) found that thought-disordered patients showed unusual semantic associations more commonly than controls, whereas non-thought-disordered patients did not.

Studies using dysphasia screening batteries

A way of detecting poor linguistic performance which is perhaps more in the spirit of the neuropsychological approach is to subject schizophrenic patients to batteries of tests designed to pick up and characterise abnormality in dysphasic patients. Three studies of this type have been carried out (DiSimoni *et al*, 1977; Faber & Reichstein, 1981; Silverberg-Shalev *et al*, 1981). In contrast to the mainly negative findings of the last group of studies, they all found that the schizophrenic patients performed significantly more poorly than normal subjects on many of the subtests.

The most illuminating of these studies is that of Faber & Reichstein (1981). They used tests from the Boston Diagnostic Aphasia Battery, additional tests of naming animals and objects, and the 'token test', which assesses syntactic competence. These were applied to schizophrenic patients diagnosed according to research criteria, who were also separated into groups with and

TABLE 9.2
Mean language test scores in schizophrenic patients with and without formal thought disorder (from Faber & Reichstein, 1981)

	Schizophrenic patients		Controls
	with FTD (n = 14)	without FTD (n = 10)	(n = 28)
Automatised sequences	7.5	7.4	7.8
Repetition of words	9.3***	9.6	9.9
Repetition of phrases	12.6*** + + +	15.1	14.9
Word reading	30.0	29.7	30.0
Responsive naming	27.2*** +	29.2	29.8
Confrontation naming	100.6	99.9	100.4
Body part naming	25.6**	26.0*	27.0
Animal naming	14.3	15.3	20.8
Picture naming	65.2**	65.9	67.5
Token test	49.3***	56.6**	59.3

*$P<0.05$, **$P<0.01$, ***$P<0.001$, schizophrenics versus controls.
+ $P<0.05$, + + + $P<0.001$, schizophrenics with formal thought disorder versus schizophrenics without formal thought disorder.

without formal thought disorder, as identified clinically by two independent raters. Their findings are shown in Table 9.2. It can be seen that the thought-disordered patients performed significantly more poorly than the controls on many of the tests, whereas the non-thought-disordered patients were not significantly impaired on most of the tests. However, it is also apparent that the magnitude of the differences was for the most part small.

In contrast to the studies of semantic, syntactic and phonemic competence described above, these studies suggest that schizophrenic patients do in fact show neurolinguistic deficits. The study of Faber & Reichstein (1981) also provides support for the view that it is patients with formal thought disorder who account for most of the abnormality. Nevertheless, the impairment in such patients is slight and does not amount to anything like a picture of dysphasia in these patients. It should be pointed out that none of the studies included a measure of overall intellectual function, and so they fail to meet the requirement of showing that language deficits in schizophrenia are present over and above any general intellectual deterioration. In fact, given the size of the differences between patients and controls, this might be the most obvious explanation of the findings.

Single case studies: the relationship to dysphasia

A respectable and currently highly fashionable method in neuropsychology is the detailed investigation of single cases showing a particular phenomenon. This approach was pioneered in schizophrenia by Chaika (1974). She subjected the speech of a single thought-disordered patient to linguistic analysis and found evidence of both semantic and syntactic abnormalities, as well as a failure to note speech errors when they occurred. She suggested that formal thought disorder might represent an intermittent and hitherto unrecognised form of dysphasia. Subsequently, Lecours & Vanier-Clement (1976) described paraphasias – erroneous substitutions of words – in schizophrenia, albeit perhaps of a qualitatively different type than those seen in dysphasia. Others (Benson, 1973; Fromkin, 1975), however, have argued against this view, taking the essentially traditional position that the abnormality in dysphasia lies in the speech mechanisms themselves, while in schizophrenia it is the thought behind the speech that is abnormal (Critchley, 1964).

The debate about the interpretation of severe schizophrenic thought disorder as a form of dysphasia goes on (Portnoff, 1982; and see Chapters 4 and 7); meanwhile there has been a single attempt to settle it empirically. Faber *et al* (1983) prepared transcripts of the speech of 14 schizophrenic patients with clearly evident formal thought disorder and 13 patients with dysphasia (fluent in 11 cases and non-fluent in 2). The transcripts were edited to remove all potential clues to diagnosis, and were then presented under blind conditions to two psychiatrists, two neurologists, and a speech pathologist (equivalent to a speech therapist in the UK). Only the speech pathologist came close to a perfect discrimination of thought-disordered schizophrenia from dysphasia, classifying 25 of the 27 transcripts correctly. The psychiatrists performed rather less well, one classifying 20 and the other classifying 22 of the transcripts correctly. Neither of the neurologists performed at greater than chance expectation. When particular psychiatric and neurological abnormalities were assessed, a certain amount of overlap between the schizophrenic and dysphasic patients was apparent. As shown in Table 9.3, a minority of the dysphasic patients were blindly rated as showing classic schizophrenic phenomena like derailment and illogicality, and one phenomenon, poverty of content of speech, was rated as present more frequently in the dysphasic than in the schizophrenic patients. Conversely, paraphasias were found to be as prevalent in the schizophrenic patients as in those with dysphasia.

Summary

Overall, the neuropsychological approach to formal thought disorder has had arguably more success than the psychological, but at the same time it has yielded somewhat paradoxical findings. On the one hand, a number of group studies have provided little evidence to suggest that schizophrenic patients, even those showing formal thought disorder, show anything more than minor linguistic abnormalities. On the other hand, the outcome of a fairly acrimonious debate on whether or not severe schizophrenic thought disorder is related to fluent dysphasia seems, from the study of Faber *et al* (1983), to have come down strongly in favour of the view that it is.

TABLE 9.3
Language abnormalities rated blindly in patients with dysphasia and schizophrenic patients with formal thought disorder (from Faber et al, 1983)

	Dysphasic patients (n = 13)	Schizophrenic patients (n = 14)	Significance of difference
Paraphasias	8	9	NS
Agrammatism	2	0	NS
Impaired comprehension of speech	5	0	$P = 0.04$
Anomia/word-finding problems	7	0	$P = 0.01$
Pronoun word problems	4	0	NS
Circumlocutions	1	0	NS
Neologisms	1	3	NS
Word approximations/idiosyncratic use of words	0	8	$P = 0.01$
Perseveration	1	4	NS
Incoherence	3	10	NS
Derailment/tangentiality	2	11	$P = 0.05$
Poverty of content	8	1	$P = 0.04$
Illogicality	1	5	NS
Clanging	0	3	NS

Conclusions

According to current thinking, the florid symptoms of schizophrenia reflect biologically determined disturbances of function at the cognitive psychological level. It seems highly likely that this explanation will ultimately be found to apply to many of the phenomena of formal thought disorder; however, the psychological studies to date have not been very successful in identifying where the dysfunction or dysfunctions might lie. Schizophrenia is also a disorder characterised by neuropsychological impairment. Studies of the neuropsychology of language have certainly revealed evidence of deficits in schizophrenic patients, but as yet there has been little to indicate that these are specific in the sense of being disproportionate to the overall level of intellectual impairment, and only slightly more to suggest that they might be seen particularly in patients with formal thought disorder.

While the separation of psychological and neuropsychological approaches to thought and language disorders in schizophrenia made at the beginning of this chapter thus seems to have yielded rather disappointing results, it is possible that bringing them together again may suggest some useful ways forward.

At the clinical level, formal thought disorder is clearly a multifaceted phenomenon, with, in all probability, different underlying psychological mechanisms operating in different patients at different times. Clinical observation also suggests that some of this heterogeneity is due to differences in its presentation in acute and chronnic patients. The stereotype of formal thought disorder in acute schizophrenia, with its rich, pseudo-philosophical and sometimes even poetic quality, is quite different from that in chronic hospitalised patients, where it often takes the form of a fragmentary, impoverished, and incoherence – the 'drivelling dementia' of Kraepelin (1913). The acute and chronic types of schizophrenia are also characterised by differing degrees of neuropsychological deficit: overall intellectual impairment is, as a rule, minor in the former, but can become moderate or marked in the latter.

Combining these two observations, it is tempting to speculate that there is a 'pure' variety of formal thought disorder which is typically seen in acute schizophrenic patients, and which is determined by unknown cognitive psychological mechanisms. This presentation is dominated by the classically described abnormalities such as derailment and poverty of content of speech; with the possible exception of neologisms, it does not resemble dysphasia in any important respects. However, with increasing severity and chronicity of illness, formal thought disorder takes on increasingly 'impure' characteristics. Here, the same underlying psychological abnormalities operate, but their expression is modified by a background of overall intellectual impairment – which must by definition involve language. If disordered thought is filtered through a linguistic apparatus which is itself defective, would it be surprising if speech became reminiscent of the speech of patients with neurological disease, and if frankly dysphasic phenomena began to intrude into the picture?

There might even be some preliminary support for such a view. Shallice *et al* (1991) applied the neuropsychological case study approach to five patients with chronic schizophrenia. Two of these showed little overall intellectual deterioration. Although these two patients exhibited specific deficits in executive function (and to a lesser extent in memory), neither of them showed any evidence of impairment on a battery of tests of language. The three other patients showed intellectual decline, severe in two. These patients all performed poorly on the language tests, and in one of them this was unexpectedly marked. When asked to identify common objects photographed from unconventional views, this patient named a glove as "an animal"; an electric iron as "a fish with a spike coming out of it . . . a jelly fish"; goggles as "octupus . . . tentacles"; a whisk as "tentacles . . . brush . . . lawnmower"; and a clarinet as "wheel support . . . man . . . animal". Shallice *et al* (1991) commented that this patient's pattern of errors was similar to that seen in patients with posterior cerebral lesions (visual associative agnosia or optic aphasia). On the other hand, it might strike psychiatrists as not dissimilar in a general sense from the style of responding displayed by some chronically hospitalised, severely thought-disordered schizophrenic patients.

References

ANDREASEN, N. C. (1979) Thought, language and communication disorders: I. Clinical assessment, definition of terms and evaluation of their reliability. *Archives of General Psychiatry*, **36**, 1315–1321.
BENSON, D. F. (1973) Psychiatric aspects of aphasia. *British Journal of Psychiatry*, **123**, 555–566.
CAMERON, N. (1939) Schizophrenic thinking in a problem-solving situation. *Journal of Mental Science*, **85**, 1012–1035.
—— (1944) Experimental analysis of schizophrenic thinking. In *Language and Thought in Schizophrenia* (ed. J. S. Kasanin). Berkeley: University of California Press.
CHAIKA, E. (1974) A linguist looks at 'schizophrenic' language. *Brain and Language*, **1**, 257–276.
—— & LAMBE, R. A. (1989) Cohesion in schizophrenic narratives, revisited. *Journal of Communication Disorders*, **22**, 407–421.
CHAPMAN, L. J. & CHAPMAN, J. P. (1973) *Disordered thought in schizophrenia*. New York: Appleton-Century-Crofts.
CRITCHLEY, M. (1964) The neurology of psychotic speech. *British Journal of Psychiatry*, **110**, 353–364.
CUTTING, J. (1985) *The Psychology of Schizophrenia*. Edinburgh: Churchill Livingstone.
DISIMONI, F. G., DARLEY, F. L. & ARONSON, A. E. (1977) Patterns of dysfunction in schizophrenic patients on an aphasia test battery. *Journal of Speech and Hearing Disorders*, **42**, 498–513.
FABER, R. & REICHSTEIN, M. B. (1981) Language dysfunction in schizophrenia. *British Journal of Psychiatry*, **139**, 519–522.
——, ABRAMS, R., TAYLOR, M. A., et al (1983) Comparison of schizophrenic patients with formal thought disorder and neurologically impaired patients with aphasia. *American Journal of Psychiatry*, **140**, 1348–1351.
FRASER, W. I., KING, K. M., THOMAS, P., et al (1986) The diagnosis of schizophrenia by language analysis. *British Journal of Psychiatry*, **148**, 275–278.
FRITH, C. D. & ALLEN, H. A. (1988) Language disorders in schizophrenia and their implications for neuropsychology. In *Schizophrenia: The Major Issues* (eds P. Bebbington & P. McGuffin). Oxford: Heinemann/Mental Health Foundation.
FROMKIN, V. (1975) A linguist looks at "A linguist looks at 'schizophrenic' language". *Brain and Language*, **2**, 498–503.
HARROW, M. & QUINLAN, D. M. (1985) *Disordered Thinking and Schizophrenic Psychopathology*. New York: Gardner Press.
HAWKS, D. V. & PAYNE, R. W. (1971) Overinclusive thought disorder and symptomatology. *British Journal of Psychiatry*, **118**, 663–670.
KRAEPELIN, E. (1913) *Dementia Praecox and Paraphrenia* (trans. R. M. Barclay, 1919). Edinburgh: Livingstone.
LECOURS, A. R. & VANIER-CLEMENT, M. (1976) Schizophasia and jargonaphasia: a comparative description with comments on Chaika's and Fromkin's respective looks at 'schizophrenic' language. *Brain and Language*, **3**, 516–565.
LIDDLE, P. F. & CROW, T. J. (1984) Age disorientation in chronic schizophrenia is associated with global intellectual impairment. *British Journal of Psychiatry*, **144**, 193–199.
MAHER, B. (1972) The language of schizophrenia: a review and interpretation. *British Journal of Psychiatry*, **120**, 3–17.
MORICE, R. & INGRAM, J. C. L. (1982) Language analysis in schizophrenia: diagnostic implications. *Australian and New Zealand Journal of Psychiatry*, **16**, 11–21.
OWENS, D. G. C. & JOHNSTONE, E. C. (1980) The disabilities of chronic schizophrenia – their nature and the factors contributing to their development. *British Journal of Psychiatry*, **136**, 384–393.
PAYNE, R. W. (1973) Cognitive abnormalities. In *Handbook of Abnormal Psychology* (ed. H. J. Eysenck). London: Pitman.
PORTNOFF, L. (1982) Schizophrenia and semantic aphasia: a clinical comparison. *International Journal of Neuroscience*, **16**, 189–197.

Rochester, S. & Martin, J. R. (1979) *Crazy Talk: A Study of The Discourse of Schizophrenic Speakers*. New York: Plenum.

Schwartz, S. (1982) Is there a schizophrenic language? *Behavioral and Brain Sciences*, **5**, 579–626.

Shallice, T., Burgess, P. W. & Frith, C. D. (1991) Can the neuropsychological case-study approach be applied to schizophrenia? *Psychological Medicine*, **21**, 661–673.

Silverberg-Shalev, R., Gordon, H. W., Bentin, S., *et al* (1981) Selective language deterioration in schizophrenia. *Journal of Neurology, Neurosurgery and Psychiatry*, **44**, 547–551.

Sims, A. (1988) *Symptoms in the Mind*. London: Baillière Tindall.

Thomas, P., King, K., Fraser, W. I., *et al* (1990) Linguistic performance in schizophrenia: a comparison of acute and chronic patients. *British Journal of Psychiatry*, **156**, 204–210.

10 Semantic processing and categorisation in schizophrenia

ERIC CHEN, PETER McKENNA and ARNOLD WILKINS

Semantic memory refers to information stored as concepts and the relationship between them (Tulving, 1983; Baddeley, 1990). The basic units of semantic information are concepts such as animals, or furniture, which are generated in the course of exposure to the environment (Ausubel, 1968; Anderson, 1980; Homa, 1984). In this process, salient features among items similar to one another are detected, and similar items are grouped together into a category. Categories reduce the complexity of incoming information, and filter redundant information (Miller, 1985; Howard, 1987). Categorisation involves deciding how well a newly presented stimulus fits into existing categories stored in memory. It has fundamental importance in determining how well an individual organism adapts to coping with a highly complex environment. Impairment of categorisation may lead to misinterpretation of the significance of environmental stimuli.

Within psychiatry, there has long been a tradition of studying categorisation in schizophrenic patients. The concept of overinclusiveness has been proposed by Cameron (1939, 1954) in relation to thought and language disorder in schizophrenia. In the original paradigm, patients were asked to sort objects into groups and Cameron noted that they exhibited "an inability to maintain the boundaries of the problem and to restrict their operations within its limits". In the following decades, there followed a proliferation of studies based on the idea of overinclusiveness. Testing paradigms evolved to include a variety of different procedures such as verbal definitions, proverb interpretations, as well as object sorting. Often, studies used a global score based on adding up scores obtained in these different procedures. Payne (1973) reviewed extensively the body of data available then, and concluded that the finding of overinclusiveness had been inconsistent and did not bear any direct relationship to the clinical phenomenon of formal thought disorder in schizophrenia.

One possible difficulty with research efforts in defining overinclusion is the lack of a clear focus on the *nature* of the information being categorised. For example, categorisation of word concepts into word concepts at a higher level (semantic categorisation) may involve a different set of cognitive processes from those involved in categorisation of unfamiliar objects into groups according to similarity in shape (object sorting).

In the last two decades, cognitive psychology has made progress in the study of the normal processes of categorisation and has refined experimental paradigms for exploring the structure of semantic memory. Several issues explored in cognitive psychology are relevant to the approach we adopted in the study reported below.

It became clear that the classic view of categorisation was untenable. This view holds that the process of deciding whether a novel item belongs to a certain category depends on a decision as to whether the item's attributes and characteristics fulfil certain defining features for the category (Millward, 1980). It was realised that it was not always possible to state explicitly a set of defining features even for some simple, common categories (Anglin, 1977). Alternative views were then considered. The prototype and the exemplar views are similar in that they propose that rather than asking for defining features, the process of categorisation involves comparison of a new item with a typical example of the category. In the case of the prototype view (e.g. Rosch, 1975, 1978; Posner & Keele, 1968, 1970), this example (the prototype) is formed by mental abstraction of previously encountered cases and may not correspond to any actual individual case. In the exemplar view (e.g. Brooks, 1978; Medin & Schaffer, 1978), the typical example is a commonly encountered item that has the best fit to the central characteristics of the category. Both views proposed that the simultaneous consideration of a large number of attributes is important in categorisation.

Another issue involves the idea that categories are organised hierarchically (Collins & Quillan, 1969). For example, the category "living things" includes 'animal' as an exemplar, 'animals' in turn includes 'birds' as an exemplar, and so on. It has been proposed that ordinarily most people deal with categories at a particular 'default' level, the so-called 'basic level' (Rosch et al, 1976). For example, 'birds' (rather than 'canary') would be a category in the basic level. In the empirical study, categories at the basic level were selected for testing.

Categories also differ in terms of how sharp or fuzzy their boundaries are (McCloskey & Glucksberg, 1978). In our study, categories with fuzzy boundaries were selected in order that the response to transition between the inside and the outside of the category could be explored.

In the huge body of empirical work on categorisation in normal people, among the most robust findings are the so-called semantic-relatedness effects (Kintsch, 1980). The time taken to make a category decision for a typical exemplar, for example *'a sparrow is a bird'*, is consistently shorter than the corresponding time for an atypical exemplar, for example *'a penguin is a bird'* (typicality effect). Similarly, the time taken to reject a related non-exemplar, for example *'an aeroplane is not a bird'*, is longer than the corresponding time for a totally unrelated non-exemplar, for example *'a diamond is not a bird'* (false-relatedness effect). Both typicality and false-relatedness effects are well replicated for normal people, and are evidence that semantic information about categories is stored in an organised fashion within memory (Chang, 1986).

The objective of our empirical study was to explore the organisation of category representations in schizophrenic patients through a similar categorisation task. A detailed description of the study and analysis of the empirical data are given by Chen *et al* (1994). This chapter focuses on the theoretical implications of the findings. A neurocomputational simulation model is proposed and its performance compared with the empirical data. For clarity and comprehensiveness, the main empirical findings are summarised.

An empirical study of categorisation in schizophrenia

Schizophrenic patients in the study were recruited from in-patient and out-patient services. Inclusion criteria comprised: Research Diagnostic Criteria for schizophrenia (Spitzer *et al*, 1978); age 20–60 years; native English speakers; normal premorbid IQ. Exclusion criteria comprised: neurological disease or head injury; drug or alcohol abuse; electroconvulsive therapy within previous year; significant impairment of eyesight.

Twenty-eight patients (18 men and 10 women, mean age 41, mean estimated premorbid IQ 109) were compared with 28 healthy volunteers (15 men and 13 women, mean age 35, mean estimated IQ 113). The two groups did not differ significantly in age, sex, or premorbid intelligence.

Each patient received a standardised assessment of clinical profile, including positive (Comprehensive Assessment of Symptom and History; Andreasen, 1987) and negative symptoms (High Royds Evaluation of Negativity; Mortimer *et al*, 1989), extrapyramidal signs and tardive dyskinesia (Simpson & Angus, 1970; Simpson *et al*, 1979), catatonic signs (Modified Rogers Scale; Lund *et al*, 1991), mood state (Montgomery–Åsberg scale; Montgomery & Åsberg, 1979), global severity (Endicott *et al*, 1976) and chronicity of illness, premorbid intelligence (National Adult Reading Test; Nelson, 1982), as well as medication dosage.

The categorisation task

Subjects were asked to decide whether an instance (e.g. chair) belonged to a category (e.g. furniture). Both the speed of responding and the nature of the response were recorded.

There were five levels of semantic-relatedness between categories and instances. For example, taking the category 'vehicle', in the *typical* condition the instance was 'bus', in the *atypical* condition the instance was 'ferry'; in the *borderline* condition the instance was 'escalator', in the *related* condition the instance was 'horse', in the *unrelated* condition the instance was 'diamond'. Forty-five such category and instance pairs were constructed out of established categorisation norms (Battig & Montague, 1969; Hampton & Gardiner, 1983). They were selected on the basis that there were no obvious affective associations. Therefore categories such as crime, weapons, diseases, and so on were not included. Words with obvious double meanings (e.g. swallow) were excluded. (The stimulus material is available upon request to EC.)

Compared with traditional categorisation paradigms, a novel feature in the current approach was the inclusion of a borderline condition (although this has been used in some studies on categorisation of visual forms). Instances (members of a category) in the borderline condition were selected on the basis that they were considered as being inside and outside the category about equally often by normal subjects. Processing time for the borderline conditions was found to be longer than in the atypical and the related conditions. The borderline condition could be considered as a rough measure of the category boundary.

Words were presented on a computer screen. The category word (e.g. furniture) appeared for two seconds and then disappeared. The instance word (e.g. chair) was presented 500 ms later. The subjects were instructed to decide whether the instance belonged to the category (emphasising accuracy rather than speed) and to respond by pressing a button. Reaction times and whether the response was 'yes' or 'no' were recorded by the computer.

Results

In the normal response pattern, reaction time for the *typical* condition was relatively short, and raised for the *atypical* condition. Reaction time was raised further in the *borderline* condition. After the category boundary was crossed, the reaction time decreased for the *related* condition and decreased further

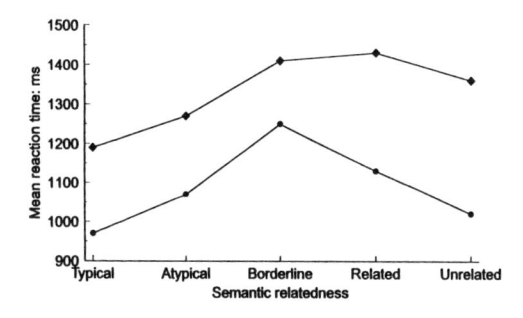

Fig. 10.1. Mean categorisation time for schizophrenic patients (♦) and controls (●) for the five conditions of different semantic relatedness (see text for details) (reprinted with permission from Psychological Medicine, *copyright 1994)*

for the *unrelated* condition (Fig. 10.1). This finding was confirmed for a further set of stimuli constructed in a similar way, indicating that the results were generalisable.

The overall speed of responding of patients was slower across all conditions. Also, the pattern of responding appeared to be different: the condition that took the longest to respond was the *related* condition, rather than the *borderline* condition (Fig. 10.1).

The data were analysed in two ways because of a degree of skewness in the reaction-time data points (more shorter reaction times). Logarithmic transformation of the reaction times approached normal distribution and were analysed with parametric methods. The second approach was to apply non-parametric methods on untransformed data. The two methods yielded similar results.

The results of analysis of variance using subject group as the between-subject variable and semantic-relatedness as the within-subject variable showed that, in addition to the effects of group – patients were slower on the whole ($F = 21.40$, d.f. $= 1, 54$, $P < 0.0001$) – and semantic-relatedness – the reaction times for the five different levels of semantic relatedness were different ($F = 40.98$, d.f. $= 4, 216$, $P < 0.0001$) – there was a significant interaction between group and condition ($F = 5.46$, d.f. $= 4, 216$, $P < 0.0003$), suggesting that the *pattern* of response across the conditions was different in patients.

To explore this difference further, analyses of variance were carried out on pairs of conditions. It was found that the interaction between group and condition was only significant between the borderline and related conditions ($F = 11.22$, d.f. $= 1, 54$, $P = 0.0015$) and not between the other conditions. This suggested that there was a qualitative difference between patients and controls in relation to the borderline and related conditions; namely, patients were having longer reaction times for the related condition.

Multiple *post hoc* pairwise comparisons using the Peritz technique (Toothaker, 1991) also confirmed this observation. In patients it was the borderline versus related, and atypical versus unrelated conditions which did *not* differ significantly (in contrast to the typical versus unrelated, and the atypical versus unrelated conditions in the controls); all other pairwise comparisons were significant at $P < 0.05$.

Apart from reaction-time data, the nature of response ('yes' or 'no') was studied. As can be seen in Fig. 10.2, patients tended to consider more instances as belonging within the category in the borderline and the related conditions.

Further analysis was carried out with an extended sample of 39 patients. No correlation was found between categorisation abnormality and chronicity of illness. Correlation analyses with symptoms were difficult because of the large number of comparisons involved. It would be interesting to see whether with a large sample size, or by identifying subgroups of patients, relationships between categorisations and symptoms might be better delineated.

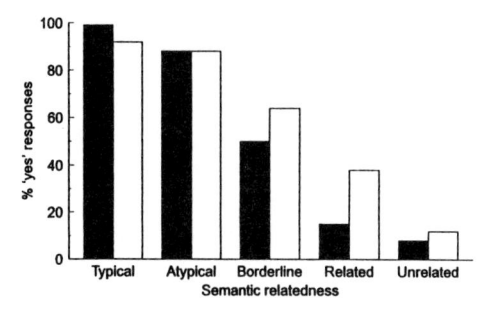

Fig. 10.2. Percentage category inclusion ('yes') responses for patients (■) and controls (□) in the five conditions of semantic relatedness (reprinted with permission from Psychological Medicine, *copyright 1994)*

Theoretical issues and computer simulation models

One immediate interpretation of the reaction-time data and the nature of responses is that schizophrenic patients are overinclusive in semantic categories. However, before considering this interpretation, several methodological issues have to be discussed.

One consideration is whether the current findings could be accounted for entirely in terms of the non-specific poor performance (due to poor motivation, a general cognitive decline, etc.) found with schizophrenic patients. There are several reasons why the current findings could not be easily accounted for by such non-specific effects. Firstly, both the typicality and false-relatedness effects are present and intact in patients. This suggests that patients were properly engaged in the task, to the level of processing required to demonstrate the semantic-relatedness effects. Secondly, the finding of an overinclusive response pattern could not simply be attributed to a lack of motivation to come to a decision and therefore responding before an appropriate threshold is reached. Such a pattern of responding should lead to shorter, not longer, reaction times in the more difficult conditions. Thirdly, the pattern of responding is unlikely to be entirely secondary to an attention deficit, as it has been shown that attention loading (by a secondary working memory task) leads to a slowing of reaction time but preservation of the normal *pattern* of responding (Baddeley *et al*, 1984).

With these considerations, one way of interpreting the findings is that in schizophrenic patients, while semantic categories have a preserved internal structure, there is an outward shift of the category boundary so that related instances, outside the category, are processed by patients in a way similar to instances inside the category boundary. In other words, the semantic categories of schizophrenic patients are overinclusive. To consider further the underlying mechanisms involved, it is necessary to review what may be the component cognitive processes involved in the categorisation task.

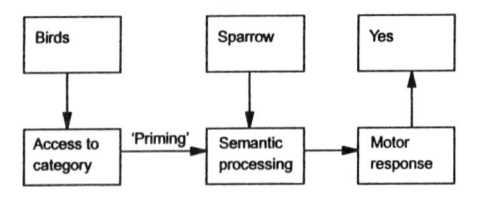

Fig. 10.3. Component processes in the categorisation task. The process labelled 'Semantic processing' compares semantic information in the instance (sparrow) with that in the category (birds). When the category is first presented, the retrieved information prepares the system for the presentation of the instance (thus creating a context, or priming). When the instance appears it is considered in the context of the category in arriving at a categorisation decision

During task performance, at least several steps of processing are likely to be involved (Fig. 10.3). Upon presentation of the category, subjects retrieve semantic information relating to the category. This information is then held in working memory in preparation for the presentation of the instance. When the instance is presented, semantic information about the instance word is retrieved and compared with that of the category, now in working memory. This comparison then leads to the category decision. Several hypotheses concerning this decision process are discussed below.

In the 'property comparison model' (McCloskey & Glucksberg, 1978), categories are represented by sets of properties. Each property is compared between the instance and the category. Positive and negative evidence accumulates in a Bayesian fashion until the probability of category inclusion or exclusion reaches a preset decision threshold.

In the 'two-stage feature comparison model' (Smith et al, 1974), two qualitatively different stages of processing are involved. In the first stage there is a global comparison between the instance and the category. If sufficient similarity is found, a positive decision is arrived at. Likewise, sufficient dissimilarity would lead to an immediate negative decision. If the comparison at this stage does not yield a decisive outcome, the second stage is entered, where defining features are considered sequentially and eventually lead to a slower decision.

Both of the above models involve some sequential processes. One potential difficulty with such processes is that the speed (and in some cases, outcome) of response may depend on the sequence in which features are compared. It is not clear how the order of sequence originates or is defined. Another difficulty with these models is the inability to account for the origin of category information in the first place. More recently, parallel-distributed (neural network or connectionist) models of mental representations have been developed (McClelland & Rumelhart, 1986). In these models, items of information are represented by patterns of activity across a large number of processing units. Changes in activity of the network with time involves and takes into account all units. Models of semantic categorisation by distributed representations are still being developed (Hinton, 1989; Anderson, 1989). A simple illustration of the approach is offered below.

A neural network simulation model

A typical distributed model consists of a large number of processing units (a 100-unit network is used in the simulation experiment) connected to one another through junctions called synapses (Fig. 10.4). The strength of each synapse is adjusted by previous exposure, according to a specified learning rule. The Hebbian rule is used in the simulation because there is evidence it may be operative in biological neural systems (e.g. Kelso *et al*, 1986; McNaughton & Morris, 1987). It states that whenever two units are active at the same time, the connection between them is strengthened; when one is active and the other is inactive, the connection is weakened.

In the learning phase, the network is exposed to repeated presentation of a number of instances, each represented by a pattern of activity distributed across all the units in the network. Synaptic strengths are modified according to which units are active in conjunction. Through this learning mechanism the network stores information about instances that it has encountered in the form of synaptic strengths. Importantly, through learning in this way networks are capable of spontaneously generating prototypes. Exposures to a number of closely related patterns could generate abstracted information about the group of patterns as a whole (thus generating a prototype from specific examples) (McClelland & Rumelhart, 1989).

Once a network is trained, it is capable of classifying novel patterns (instances) into existing stored patterns (categories). When a novel pattern is encountered, the network starts with a pattern of activity corresponding to the novel pattern. From this initial state of activity, the network evolves according to internal constraints. In each time-step, each processing unit in the network changes its level of activation according to the activation of

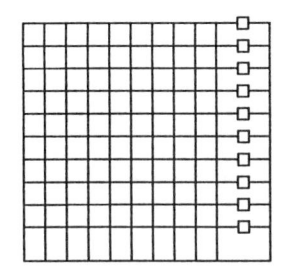

Fig. 10.4. An auto-associative network consists of a number of processing units (blank squares). Each unit has a level of activation. The output of the units (lines to the right) is connected via 'synapses' (intersection of lines) with input lines (to the left of the units) of all other units in the network. The level of activation of a unit at a particular time-step is a function of its previous activation and the current input. The input is itself a function of the activation of connected units and the strength of the connection

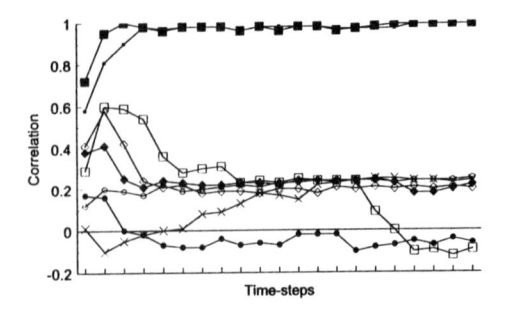

Fig. 10.5. Behaviour of a neural network modelling categorisation processes. Initial patterns at time-step = 0 (examplars) correlate to the prototype to differing extents (correlation: number of units in pattern being in the same state as corresponding units in prototype). When the network is presented with these patterns (one at a time) it evolves in different manners. Initial patterns of high correlation (typical) (initial correlation greater than 0.7) lead to a fast positive decision. Slightly less correlated patterns (atypical) (initial correlation between 0.4 and 0.7) settles with a slower positive decision. Low-correlation (related) patterns (initial correlation between 0.3 and 0.4) settle to a slow negative decision. Uncorrelated (unrelated) patterns (initial correlation less than 0.2) result in quick negative decisions. Category boundary is between correlation of 0.4 and 0.6

other units in the network and the strength of connection with these units. In this way information previously stored in synaptic connections gradually guide the network to 'settle' into a pattern of activity corresponding to, or close to, a previously learned pattern. Categorisation processes may be modelled by such settling of the network state from an initial pattern (instance) to the final pattern (category) (Fig. 10.5).

'Priming' refers to the facilitation in recognition of a word presented subsequently to the presentation of a semantically related word. Evidence for an excessive priming has been reported in schizophrenic patients (Manschreck et al, 1988; Chapin et al, 1989; Kwapil et al, 1990; Spitzer, 1992). Using our simple distributed model, the relationship between excessive priming and categorisation processes in schizophrenic patients is represented by introducing a computational equivalent of excessive priming for the category pattern (by lowering its threshold for activation). In this situation, simulation experiment demonstrates that borderline instances now lead to a positive decision. An instance previously leading to a negative decision (related condition) now hovers in the region of indecision, and may lead to an eventual positive response after a longer latency (resembling the borderline condition). Previous borderline patterns (positive or negative decision after very long latency) are now treated as if they are within the category and a positive decision is made after a long latency (resembling the atypical condition) (Fig. 10.6). This 'overinclusive' pattern of response is similar to the responses made by schizophrenic patients in the empirical study.

Although only a simple illustrative device, the network model offers several features not available in the conventional sequential models (being able to account for the origin of prototypes and processing of global information

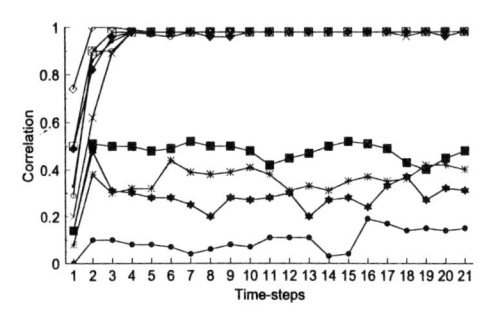

Fig. 10.6. Categorisation behaviour of a network 'primed' for the prototype pattern (threshold lowered by 10%). Patterns of relatively low correlation (0.3) still lead to slow positive decisions (related-condition response similar to borderline condition). Category boundary between 0.2–0.3

at each time-step), and it suggests a way of relating the current finding of overinclusiveness in semantic categorisation to excessive semantic priming found in lexical decision tasks.

Conclusions

A categorisation task is a method of exploring the structure of semantic memory in schizophrenia. Empirical data suggest that in schizophrenic patients semantic categories are intact internally, but the category boundaries are expanded. A simple parallel-distributed model is able to accommodate findings from the study and link these to recent findings of excessive semantic priming in schizophrenia. It is hoped that the data would invite further speculations as to the cognitive processes involved, such as the interaction between working memory and semantic memory in categorisation, and the extent to which these processes are affected in psychosis. Further studies are required to delineate their relationship with psychopathology and possible neurobiological processes.

References

ANDERSON, J. A. (1989) Categorization and selective neurons. In *Parallel Models of Associative Memory* (eds G. E. Hinton & J. A. Anderson), pp. 251–274. Hillsdale: Lawrence Erlbaum.
ANDERSON, J. R. (1980) *Cognitive Psychology and its Implications*. San Francisco: Freeman.
ANDREASEN, N. C. (1987) *The Comprehensive Assessment of Symptoms and History*. Iowa City: University of Iowa College of Medicine.
ANGLIN, J. M. (1977) *Word, Object and Conceptual Development*. New York: Norton.
AUSUBEL, D. P. (1968) *Educational Psychology: A Cognitive View*. New York: Holt, Rinehart and Winston.
BADDELEY, A. (1990) *Human Memory: Theory and Practice*. Hillsdale: Lawrence Erlbaum.
——, LEWIS, V., ELDRIDGE, M., *et al* (1984) Attention and retrieval from long-term memory. *Journal of Experimental Psychology: General*, **113**, 518–540.

BATTIG, W. F. & MONTAGUE, W. E. (1969) Category norms for verbal items in 56 categories: a replication and extension of the Connecticut category norms. *Journal of Experimental Psychology (Monograph)*, **80**, 1-45.

BROOKS, L. (1978) Non-analytic concept formation and memory for instances. In *Cognition and Categorisation* (eds E. Rosch & B. B. Lloyd). Hillsdale: Lawrence Erlbaum.

CAMERON, N. (1939) Schizophrenic thinking in a problem-solving situation. *Journal of Mental Science*, **85**, 1012-1035.

—— (1954) Experimental analysis of schizophrenic thinking. In *Language and Thought in Schizophrenia* (ed. J. S. Kasanin), pp. 50-63. Berkeley: University of California Press.

CHANG, T. M. (1986) Semantic memory: facts and models. *Psychological Bulletin*, **99**, 199-220.

CHAPIN, K., VANN, L. E., LYCAKI, H., et al (1989) Investigation of the associative network in schizophrenia using the semantic priming paradigm. *Schizophrenia Research*, **2**, 355-360.

CHEN, E. Y. H., WILKINS, A. J. & MCKENNA, P. J. (1994) Semantic memory is both impaired and anomalous in schizophrenia. *Psychological Medicine*, **24**, 193-202.

COLLINS, A. M. & QUILLIAN, M. R. (1969) Retrieval time from semantic memory. *Journal of Verbal Learning and Verbal Behaviour*, **8**, 240-248.

—— & LOFTUS, E. F. (1975) A spreading-activation theory of semantic processing. *Psychological Review*, **82**, 407-428.

ENDICOTT, J., SPITZER, R. C., FLIESS, J. L., et al (1976) The global assessment scale. *Archives of General Psychiatry*, **33**, 766-771.

HAMPTON, J. A. & GARDINER, M. M. (1983) Measures of internal category structure: a correlational analysis of normative data. *British Journal of Psychology*, **74**, 491-516.

HINTON, G. E. (1989) Implementing semantic networks in parallel hardware. In *Parallel Models of Associative Memory* (eds G. E. Hinton & J. A. Anderson), pp. 191-217. Hillsdale: Lawrence Erlbaum.

HOMA, D. (1984) On the nature of categories. In *The Psychology of Learning and Motivation, Vol. 18* (ed. G. H. Bower). New York: Academic Press.

HOWARD, R. W. (1987) *Concepts and Schemata: An Introduction*. London: Cassell Educational.

KELSO, S. R., GANONG, A. H. & BROWN, T. H. (1986) Hebbian synapses in hippocampus. *Proceedings of the National Academy of Sciences, USA*, **83**, 5326-5330.

KINTSCH, W. (1980) Semantic memory: a tutorial. In *Attention and Performance VIII* (ed. R. S. Nickerson), pp. 595-620. Hillsdale: Lawrence Erlbaum.

KWAPIL, T. R., HEGLEY, D. C., CHAPMAN, L. J., et al (1990) Facilitation of word recognition by semantic priming in schizophrenia. *Journal of Abnormal Psychology*, **99**, 215-221.

LUND, C. E., MORTIMER, A. M., MCKENNA, P. J., et al (1991) Motor, volitional and behavioural disorders in schizophrenia: (I) Assessment using the modified Rogers scale. *British Journal of Psychiatry*, **158**, 323-327.

MANSCHRECK, T. C., MAHER, B. A., MILAVETZ, J. J., et al (1988) Semantic priming in thought disordered schizophrenic patients. *Schizophrenia Research*, **1**, 61-66.

MCCLELLAND, J. & RUMELHART, D. E. (1986) *Parallel Distributed Processing: Explorations in the Microstructure of Cognition. Volume 2: Psychological and Biological Models*. Cambridge, MA: MIT Press.

—— & —— (1989) *Explorations in Parallel Distributed Processing*. Cambridge, MA: MIT Press.

MCCLOSKEY, M. E. & GLUCKSBERG, S. (1978) Natural categories: well-defined or fuzzy sets? *Memory and Cognition*, **6**, 642-672.

—— & —— (1979) Decision processes in verifying category membership statements: implications for models of semantic memory. *Cognitive Psychology*, **11**, 1-37.

MCNAUGHTON, B. L. & MORRIS, R. G. (1987) Hippocampal synaptic enhancement and information storage within a distributed memory system. *Trends in Neuroscience*, **10**, 408-415.

MEDIN, D. L. & SCHAFFER, M. M. (1978) Context theory of classification learning. *Psychological Review*, **85**, 207-238.

MILLER, G. A. (1985) Trends and debates in cognitive psychology. In *Issues in Cognitive Modeling* (eds A. M. Aitkenhead & J. M. Slack), pp. 3-12. London: Lawrence Erlbaum.

MILLWARD, R. B. (1980) Models of concept formation. In *Aptitude, Learning and Instruction: Cognitive Process Analyses of Learning and Problem Solving* (eds R. E. Snow, P. Federico & W. E. Montague). Hillsdale: Lawrence Erlbaum.

MONTGOMERY, S. A. & ÅSBERG, M. (1979) A new depression scale designed to be sensitive to change. *British Journal of Psychiatry*, **139**, 382–389.
MORTIMER, A. M., LUND, C. E. & MCKENNA, P. J. (1989) Rating of negative symptoms using the HEN scale. *British Journal of Psychiatry*, **155** (suppl. 7), 89–92.
NELSON, H. E. (1982) *The National Adult Reading Test (NART)*. Windsor: NFER-Nelson.
PAYNE, R. W. (1973) Cognitive abnormalities. In *Handbook of Abnormal Psychology* (ed. H. J. Eysenck), pp. 420–483. London: Pitman.
POSNER, M. I. & KEELE, S. W. (1968) On the genesis of abstract ideas. *Journal of Experimental Psychology*, **77**, 353–363.
—— & —— (1970) Retention of abstract ideas. *Journal of Experimental Psychology*, **83**, 304–308.
ROSCH, E. (1975) Cognitive representation of semantic categories. *Journal of Experimental Psychology: General*, **104**, 192–233.
—— (1978) Principles of categorisation. In *Cognition and Categorisation* (eds E. Rosch & B. B. Lloyd). Hillsdale: Lawrence Erlbaum.
——, MERVIS, C. B., GRAY, W. D., et al (1976) Basic objects in natural categories. *Cognitive Psychology*, **8**, 382–439.
SIMPSON, G. M. & ANGUS, J. W. S. (1970) Drug induced extrapyramidal disorders. *Acta Psychiatrica Scandinavica* (suppl. 212), 1–58.
——, LEE, J. H., ZOUBOK, B., et al (1979) A rating scale for tardive dyskinesia. *Psychopharmacology*, **64**, 171–179.
SMITH, E. E., SHOBEN, E. J. & RIPS, L. J. (1974) Structure and process in semantic memory: a featural model for semantic decisions. *Psychological Review*, **81**, 214–241.
SPITZER, M. (1992) Word-associations in experimental psychiatry: a historical perspective. In *Phenomenology, Language and Schizophrenia* (eds M. Spitzer, F. Uchlein, M. A. Schwartz, et al), pp. 160–169. New York: Springer-Verlag.
SPITZER, R. L., ENDICOTT, J. & ROBINS, E. (1978) *Research Diagnostic Criteria for a Selected Group of Functional Disorders*. New York: New York State Psychiatric Institute.
TOOTHAKER, L. (1991) *Multiple Comparisons for Researchers*. California: Sage.
TULVING, E. (1983) *Elements of Episodic Memory*. Oxford: Oxford University Press.

11 German concepts of schizophrenic language disorder and reality assessment

CHRISTOPH MUNDT

Schizophrenia research in Germany has shifted its focus during the past 20 years from the patient in the social environment to the organic basis of abnormal phenomena. Neuroanatomical studies, genetics, and cognitive neuroscience have succeeded social psychiatric approaches and the so-called 'anthropological phenomenology' which flourished in particular in the Heidelberg school in the 1950s and 1960s. The same applies to research into thought and language disturbances. After the initial association studies by Kraepelin (1896), Aschaffenburg (1896, 1899), and Bleuler (1911) (see Spitzer, 1993), there followed a period characterised by careful clinical descriptions (e.g. Berze & Gruhle, 1929). Then the interest subsided. Kurt Schneider (1974) did not mention language and speech disturbances among the first-rank symptoms. In the 1960s, anthropological phenomenology discovered speech and language disorders as a model for schizophrenia. Nowadays linguistic methods are more appealing because of their objective, quantitative nature.

This chapter examines some of the psychopathological observations and hypotheses of those decades from the end of the 1950s until the early 1970s, when anthropological phenomenology had taken the lead in German psychopathology. Apart from the historical interest, this will serve to draw attention to what may be called the 'psychonomian' level of pathogenesis in speech and language disorders. The term 'psychonomy' signifies meaningful connections within a person's mental set up (e.g. motives), as well as stages of decomposition and repair of mental function in a functional as opposed to organic sense. As with cognitive neuroscience – especially neural network modelling (Kosslyn & Koenig, 1992) – this approach does not involve the investigation of the material basis of these functions (unlike the neuroanatomical theories which considered schizophrenic speech and language disturbances as a variant of aphasias and paraphasias). In general, the approach to the psychonomian realm of these phenomena works with what Karl Jaspers (1965) called 'comprehending psychopathology' rather than experimental techniques.

Before discussing schizophrenic language disorders from the point of view of those who adopted 'comprehending psychopathology', it is necessary first to look at normal language functions, and how they may be disturbed.

Normal speech and language functions and their disturbance

The most obvious aspect of normal speech is the transmission of information. Glatzel (1978) introduced a view of schizophrenic language disturbances which focused on this aspect. For successful communication, according to Glatzel, the context of the communicative action has to be defined by means of 'metacommunication' (e.g. the situation of the psychiatric interview). Glatzel called its disturbance 'interactional psychopathology' to take into consideration the role of the interviewer. Symbolic interactionism as well as theories about the act of speech served as theoretical background.

Joachim Küchenhoff (1991) resumed this approach recently by adopting a classification system of speech acts developed by Jürgen Habermas, the philosopher of the so-called 'Frankfurt Critical School'. Habermas (1981) considered the agreement between the communication partners on the definition of the situation as the aim of speaking. If agreement is obtained, the speaker then develops and asserts a set of meanings, a procedure which Habermas called 'illocution'. The speaker is not requested to tell the truth but to be authentic; subjectivity is to be established, not objectivity. Habermas derived four types of distorted communication. First was fading of the illocutive strength, which Küchenhoff parallels to negative language disturbances in schizophrenia. Second was the speaker's inability to restrict the applicability of illocution, as for example in incorrect generalisations. Third was mistaking different areas of applicability of illocution, as for example in concretism or in misperception of the metaphorical level. Fourth was the inability to act according to the agreement in dialogue.

Although this system was not primarily developed to describe psychopathological deviance, it seems to be applicable to the deviant speech of schizophrenic patients. Nevertheless, theories of speech acts have one disadvantage: they are oriented too closely to scientific discourse, and tend to disregard affective components.

Speech competence is but one aspect of normal thinking and language. Blankenburg (1976, 1984, 1991) pointed out that, paradoxically, lack of language ability is as important as competence, in the sense that modes of expression have to be found to say the inexpressible. All languages seem to have several expressions for being dumbfounded. Thus, Blankenburg focuses on the tension between the inexpressible in preverbal thinking on one side and the strait-jacket of predicative, everyday language for representing reality on the other side. Normal thinking and speaking moves in circular fashion between these areas. Kleist, for example, in the

18th century demonstrated this in his essay on elaborating thoughts while speaking. Blankenburg assumes a constant struggle for adequate expression of preverbal contents. Language seems to have the tendency to proceed from the vague, pre-predicative contents of feelings, of atmosphere, or of a state of mind, to concrete terms as representations of the world and to falsifiable judgements. For some purposes this precision can be a nuisance, although it is strived for in scientific discourse. Poetry tries to dwell on these pre-predicative roots of language, even tries actively to avoid being taken too concretely (as with the language of music). The creativity of schizophrenic artists has its roots in this preponderance of pre-predicative thinking. This tension and the continual attempt to find adequate expression is, according to Blankenburg, a strong argument against Whorf's language relativism, which denies the possibility of thinking and expressing oneself beyond a given language.

Another example of this necessary openness to preverbal impressions is the fact that language is permanently renewed. After years of use, metaphors and sayings lose their authenticity, and a new language has to be created to narrow the gap again between the impressionistic pre-predicative mode of thinking and preformed pathways of thinking. Blankenburg compares this relation – worn-out language – novel modes of expressing feelings – with the figure–background relationship in terms of Gestalt psychology.

Another example is the language of adolescents, with their provoking use of taboo words, which cleans the language of the dust of conventions.

What is essential for this aspect of language is the unfinalised character of producing meaning in language, the necessity of a permanent struggle for adequate expression in order to narrow the gap between preverbal feeling or thinking and the precision of predicative language. It is in exactly this moving back and forth between preverbal and verbal thinking where Blankenburg localises schizophrenic disturbance of thought and language.

There is a wide field of philosophical conceptualisations of those mental acts which bring about these steps of thinking. The culmination of this philosophy of intentionality is represented by Husserl. Michael Schwartz, O. P. Wiggins and F. A. Uehlein have provided new attempts to apply it to the psychopathology of schizophrenia (Wiggins *et al*, 1990; Mundt, 1990*a*; Uehlein, 1992*a,b*).

Probably the most basic use of language is to cause a specific action in the listener. This it does with the pre-predicative mode of communication. Ethological studies describe precisely defined signals by which, for example, a flight of crows is started. A barking or whining dog may intend to deter somebody if scared, or evade punishment. A crying infant may induce feeding. All these utterances are near to the somatic substrate in the sense that they are genetically fairly well defined, as Konrad Lorenz (1965) demonstrated, and that they are combined with non-verbal elements of communication. Modern interpretations of delusion as concretism centre on these pre-predicative utterances inducing a certain behaviour. Tress & Pfaffenberger (1991), Glatzel (1978), and Spitzer (1989) consider this as the essential characteristic of delusional communication: the patient defines the communication as though it were predicative, but it is in fact pre-predicative and thus signifies the mental condition of the speaker, which cannot be falsified – it is not a judgement subject to agreement.

Self-presentation and representation of the speaker in the communication, simply to get in touch and not necessarily to make a statement, is another anthropological category of language, as Kraus (1991) pointed out. According to the structuralists Peters (1973, 1978) and Lang (1982, 1991), this act ultimately is bound to an intact subjectivity without dissolved ego boundaries or merging into another individual (dyadic fusion). Peters (1981) illustrates this aspect of language by describing the impersonal character of the late Hölderlin's language, which is almost completely devoid of personal pronouns, especially 'I' and 'me'.

Another aspect of language is its possible religious character, for example oaths, curses, confessions, and absolutions. Dörr-Zegers (1991) drew a parallel between religious revelation and misperceptions of word meaning, delusional perception, or creation of neologism by schizophrenic patients. Concretism and reification of words and phrases can be considered as resting on this magic power of naming things.

Some examples of German phenomenological approaches to schizophrenic speech and language disturbance

Peters (1973) observed circumscribed misperceptions of a single word or single sentence by schizophrenic patients which prevented their being understood. These patients showed no further language or thought disturbance, but were unable to correct their misperception, even after an explanation. Peters called this circumscribed disturbance of the semantics of a single word or single sentence 'sign-field disturbance'. He broadened this observation to include the situational context in which the misperception happened, stating that the science of literature rather than of linguistics has to be applied. The most difficult situations involved the patients affirming themselves, particularly if this had to happen in opposition to the expectations or suppositions of a significant other person.

To illustrate this paradigm, the case is described of a patient who produced schizophasic speech at a certain point in the interview (Mundt, 1988).

Case example

The patient was referred to the out-patient department for an opinion because she had shown some bizarre behaviour after a traffic accident she had caused. The woman, in her mid-30s, had already been assessed some weeks before and had been considered healthy. Apart from a vague 'praecox' feeling (in the sense of Rümke), no psychopathological symptoms were found in two sessions. In these sessions, as well as in the previous reference, the interview consisted of clear-cut questions and fairly short answers. When reaching a point within the biographical anamnesis, where the patient had experienced a failure in her professional life and eventually had been dismissed from her company, her utterances became more vague. So she was asked to talk about this topic for 10 minutes without interruption and without further questions. The patient agreed to have her talk recorded. The severely schizophasic talk which then developed (which is unfortunately untranslatable) and which instantly clarified the diagnosis can be interpreted with regard to the emotional structure of the situation. The patient felt embarassed and called upon to justify herself because of the disruption in her work record, as she had been very ambitious. Moreover, she was under the threat of being fined because of the traffic accident, and she was afraid to be admitted for a psychiatric illness because this would disrupt her very autistic, probably self-protective life. On the other hand, treatment and care were being offered to her. The patient was therefore tense and undecided on what to say and how to present herself. The difference between this interview, in which her disorder became apparent, and the previous two, in which she appeared healthy, was only in the open, 10-minute explanation to the interviewer, under great emotional pressure, with little structure, and in an ambiguous social situation. This is exactly the condition, described by several qualitative studies in German psychopathology, which frequently precipitates decompensation of a schizophrenic patient's intentional efforts (cf. Kisker, 1960).

Lang (1982) studied 15 hebephrenic patients in long-term psychotherapy. He described a 'pernicious fusion' of these patients with their mothers, accompanied by the psychological absence of the father. Lang found that these patients got stuck in the dyadic relationship with their mother in adolescence, and thus were unable to take social roles outside these dyadic relationships. Some of these patients developed a delusional attempt to identify with father figures at the beginning of the psychosis. Lang interpreted his findings, under the influence of Jacques Lacan's structuralism, as a lack of the patient's symbolisation of primordial relationships. According to Lacan's and Lang's theory, affects, feelings and impulses need representation in symbols, otherwise they cannot be distanced, tamed, or handled. The human world of imaginations, desires and fears is bound to this representational mode. Distance from the mother by symbolic representation is the premise for freeing oneself from the prison of immediate, unsymbolised desires and fears. Only if symbolisation is brought about can a separate self be constituted, and the dyadic relationship can become triadic, which includes the father as a representative of external reality. French psychiatry makes the same point by talking of the missing 'third pole' in conversation with schizophrenic patients. 'Third pole' describes the need for the dyadic conversation to obey the body of semantic meanings of the social community to which the speakers belong.

Janzarik is another German psychopathologist who has proposed a theory of speech and language disorders. His work may be considered as a link between phenomenology and empirical research. Janzarik (1988) discusses schizophrenic thought and language disorders from the viewpoint of his structural–dynamic anthropology. In his view, continuity of psychic dynamism and the specific human world of experiences, feelings, and thoughts is necessarily bound to the representational mode of affects. In this respect he agrees with the structuralists, Peters and Lang. According to Janzarik, dealing with reality as mediated by representations needs more mental effort than dealing with what is immediately experienced. Schizophrenic people have difficulties in sustaining and 'bringing home' intentions on a metaphorical level. Janzarik presumes an insufficiency of the basic personality dynamism in schizophrenic people to be the cause of this phenomenon, in conjunction with difficulties with overobtrusive mental contents. These observations, and their conceptualisations derived from the clinical phenomena of acute and chronic psychoses, fit very well with the experimental work of some younger authors of the Heidelberg school, such as Holm-Hadulla on concretism, and Spitzer on the activational states of associative networks in schizophrenia.

In a controlled study, Holm-Hadulla *et al* (1991) investigated the ability of patients with schizophrenia to interpret proverbs. He used operationalised criteria for substituting the concrete meaning of the proverb by an abstract statement, for transferring the point the proverb makes to human life, and for 'intermingling' (a criterion suggested by Harrow to register personalising and bizarre interpretations which are coloured by the patients' conflicts). The authors found clear differences on substitution and transference with better performance of the control group, while 'intermingling' was similar in the two groups. In interpreting these results, Holm-Hadulla refers to Goldstein & Scheerer's (1947) term 'concretism' to explain the patients' overexclusion and general uncertainty in dealing with changing levels of metaphorical abstraction. Overabstraction is as well observed as concretism; concretism and abstraction both lead to a failure to arrive at the intended metaphorical level. There is similar evidence of a missing metaphorical level in the paintings and sculptures of schizophrenic artists. For example, in the paintings of Richard Dadd any allegory is blurred or mistaken, so that the painting is difficult if not impossible to interpret, although brilliant in technique. Similar phenomena can be observed in art objects of the Heidelberg Prinzhorn Collection (Mundt, 1990*b*).

There is yet another level of mental life in which the schizophrenic subject's difficulty with meaning and purpose becomes manifest. In a study on intentional contents and qualities of striving in the life histories of psychiatric patients, it could be shown (Mundt & Becker, 1995) that schizophrenic patients develop less clear-cut 'themes for striving in adolescence' than depressives and neurotic patients.

The philosophers' 'ontologisation' of language, as Blankenburg (1991) put it, seems to be a concretism itself, since the observed phenomena are found on all levels of the schizophrenic person's self-explication, not only on the language level. What all the concepts have in common is the assumption that the patient has difficulties in moving back and forth between the vague, sensual, preverbal feelings, and the predicative level of talking, painting, thinking, or acting. All theoretical constructs try to grasp this psychopathological core of schizophrenia.

The most recent approach to language disturbances in schizophrenia in German psychopathology is, again, being pursued by a Heidelberg researcher, Spitzer (1993). He uses the semantic priming paradigm in order to prove Maher's (1972) hypothesis of activated or disinhibited semantic associations in acutely thought-disordered schizophrenic patients. Semantic priming (see Chapter 10), especially indirect (with words semantically more distant to the target word) rather than direct, distinguishes thought-disordered patients, from non-thought-disordered patients and from normal subjects. In thought-disordered patients, associations spread faster and further through the associative network. Thus the stimulus word and final word appear to be more obliquely related to each other than in the more restricted and confined associative oscillations of normal and non-thought-disordered schizophrenic subjects. Clinically, this may be interpreted as evidence that what is planned – the intended contents – and what is actually uttered by the patient are discrepant because words only obliquely related to the intended meaning become active and are used. By this method the state of activation of the associative network can be characterised. The influence of different biological variables (e.g. the dopamine system) on the activational state of the network can be tested. With this model Spitzer has taken up Bleuler's old association research with modern, computer-based techniques. Perhaps this paradigm will be able to narrow the gap between the patient and the technical/instrumental aspects of mental life, between command and executive.

Conclusions

German psychopathological work on schizophrenic thought and language disturbances in the last 40 years does not view such disorders as isolated symptoms, but puts them into the broader frame of disturbed individuation and disturbed 'intersubjectivity'. This requires an analysis of the communicative constellation in which thought and language disturbances arise. The representational mode of affects and real things is accepted by all authors. However, the structuralists' assumption that the structure of language cannot be 'trespassed' (in the sense of language relativism) is questioned by others. They assume that language and thinking are just one field of psychic phenomena where the schizophrenic person's inability to achieve clarity of meaning and purpose can manifest.

The group of authors introduced here splits into two generations. The younger ones adopt more objective, empirical methods. At present, computer modelling of neural networks seems to be most promising. However, progress in gaining knowledge and in understanding the nature of schizophrenic disturbance needs to relate to past research on the psychonomian level, even if it does seem speculative to us now.

References

ASCHAFFENBURG, G. (1896) Experimentelle Studien über Associationen I. In *Psychologische Arbeiten Vol. I* (ed. E. Kraepelin), pp. 209–299. Leipzig: Engelmann.
—— (1899) Experimentelle Studien über Associationen II. In *Psychologische Arbeiten Vol. II* (ed. E. Kraepelin), pp. 1–83. Leipzig: Engelmann.
BERZE, J. & GRUHLE, H. W. (1929) *Psychologie der Schizophrenie*. Berlin: Springer.
BLANKENBURG, W. (1976) Zur Abwandlung der Funktion der Sprache bei Schizophrenen. In *Die Sprache des Anderen* (eds G. Hofer & K. P. Kisker), pp. 111–117. Basel: Karger.
—— (1984) Störungen von Auffassung und Sprache bei Schizophrenen. In *Sprache–Sprechen–Verstehen* (eds H. J. Bochnik & W. Richtberg), pp. 104–115. Erlangen: Perimed.
—— (1991) Über das Verhältnis Schizophrener zur Sprache – sprachlicher und vorsprachlicher Realitätsbezug. In *Schizophrenie und Sprache* (eds A. Kraus & Ch. Mundt), pp. 140–151. Stuttgart: Thieme.
BLEULER, E. (1911) *Dementia Praecox: Or the Group of Schizophrenias*. New York: International University Press.
DÖRR-ZEGERS, O. (1991) Die Destruktion von Sprache zur schizophrenen ''Logopathie''. In *Schizophrenie und Sprache* (eds A. Kraus & Ch. Mundt), pp. 97–104. Stuttgart: Thieme.
GLATZEL, J. (1978) *Allgemeine Psychopathologie*. Stuttgart: Enke.
GOLDSTEIN, K. & SCHEERER, M. (1947) *Abstract and Concrete Behaviour*. Evanston: American Psychological Association.
HABERMAS, J. (1981) *Theorie des Kommunikativen Handelns*. Frankfurt: Suhrkamp.
HOLM-HADULLA, H., BENZENHÖFER, U. & ROSCHMANN, R. (1991) Zur Struktur schizophrenen Denkens und Sprechens – eine mittels Sprichwortinterpetationen empirisch fundierte psychopathologische Perspektive. In *Schizophrenie und Sprache* (eds A. Kraus & Ch. Mundt), pp. 61–70. Stuttgart: Thieme.
JANZARIK, W. (1988) Strukturdynamische Grundlagen der Psychiatrie. Stuttgart: Enke.
JASPERS, K. (1965) *Allgemeine Psychopathologie*. Heidelberg: Springer. (*General Psychopathology* (trans. J. Hoenig & G. W. Henry, 1963). Manchester: Manchester University Press.)
KISKER, K. P. (1960) *Der Erlebniswandel des Schizophrenen. Ein psychopathologischer Beitrag zur Psychonomie schizophrener Grundsituationen*. Berlin: Springer.
KOSSLYN, S. M. & KOENIG, O. (1992) *Wet Mind. The New Cognitive Neuroscience*. New York: Free Press.
KRAEPELIN, E. (1896) Der psychologische Versuch in der Psychiatrie. In *Psychologische Arbeiten Vol. I* (E. Kraepelin), pp. 1–91. Leipzig: Engelmann.
KRAUS, A. (1991) Zur Topologie schizophrener Denk- und Sprachstörungen im Wesen der Sprache. In *Schizophrenie und Sprache* (eds A. Kraus & Ch. Mundt), pp. 3–7. Stuttgart: Thieme.
KÜCHENHOFF, J. (1991) Psychische Abnormität als Störung kommunikativer Kompetenz. In *Schizophrenie und Sprache* (eds A. Kraus & Ch. Mundt), pp. 53–60. Stuttgart: Thieme.
LANG, H. (1982) Struktural-analytische Gesichtspunkte zum Verständnis der schizophrenen Psychose. In *Psychopathologische Konzepte der Gegenwart* (ed. W. Janzarik), pp. 150–157. Stuttgart: Enke.
—— (1991) Verdrängung und Spaltung. Überlegungen zur Grenzziehung zwischen Neurose und Psychose im Ausgang von einem linguistisch-strukturalen Ansatz. In *Schizophrenie und Sprache* (eds A. Kraus & Ch. Mundt), pp. 90–96. Stuttgart: Thieme.

LORENZ, K. (1965) *Über tierisches und menschliches Verhalten. Aus dem Werdegang der Verhaltenslehre.* Vol. I, II. München: Piper.

MAHER, B. A. (1972) The language of schizophrenia: a review and interpretation. *British Journal of Psychiatry*, **120**, 4–17.

MUNDT, CH. (1988) Zur intentionalen Struktur einer schizophasischen Selbstdarstellung. In *Psychopathology and Philosophy* (eds M. Spitzer & F. A. Uehlein), pp. 85–95. Heidelberg: Springer.

—— (1990a) Concepts of intentionality and their application to the psychopathology of schizophrenia – a critique of the vulnerability model. In *Philosophy and Psychopathology* (eds M. Spitzer & B. Maher), pp. 35–44. New York: Springer.

—— (1990b) Über Leben und Werk von Richard Dadd – Anmerkungen zur Pathographie eines geisteskranken Malers. In *Melancholie in Literatur und Kunst* (eds D. v. Engelhardt, H.-J. Gerigk, G. Pressler & W. Schmitt), pp. 127–161. Hürtgenwald: Pressler.

—— & BECKER, E. (1995) Inhalte und Verlaufsweisen des Strebens in der Lebensgeschichte psychiatrischer Patienten. Vorläufige Ergebnisse. *Fundamenta Psychiatrica* (in press).

PETERS, U. H. (1973) Wortfeld-Störung und Satzfeld-Störung. *Archiv für Psychiatrische Nervenkrank*, **217**, 1–10.

—— (1978) Einführung in eine strukturale Psychopathologie. *Z. Klinische Psychiatrische Psychotherapie*, **26**, 5–22.

—— (1981) Hölderlin: Dichter, Kranker – Simulant? *Nervenarzt*, **52**, 261–268.

SCHNEIDER, K. (1974) Primary and secondary symptoms in schizophrenia. *Fortschritte Neurologie und Psychiatrie*, **25**, 487–490. (Trans. H. Marshall. In *Themes and Variations in European Psychiatry* (eds S. R. Hirsch & M. Sheperd). Bristol: John Wright.)

SPITZER, M. (1989) *Was ist Wahn? Untersuchungen zum Wahnproblem*. Heidelberg: Springer.

—— (1993) Assoziative Netzwerke, formale Denkstörungen und Schizophrenie. Zur experimentellen Psychopathologie sprachunabhängiger Denkprozesse. *Nervenarzt*, **64**, 147–159.

——, UEHLEIN, F., SCHWARTZ, M. A., et al (eds) (1992) *Phenomenology, Language, and Schizophrenia*: New York: Springer.

TRESS, W. & PFAFFENBERGER, U. (1991) Die sprachliche Verwendung des Begriffs "schizophren". In *Schizophrenie und Sprache* (eds A. Kraus & Ch. Mundt), pp. 38–52. Stuttgart: Thieme.

UEHLEIN, F. A. (1992a) Eidos and eidetic variation in Husserl's phenomenology. In *Phenomenology, Language, and Schizophrenia* (eds M. Spitzer *et al*), pp. 88–102. New York: Springer.

—— (1992b) Phenomenology: intentionality, passive synthesis, and primary consciousness. In *Phenomenology, Language, and Schizophrenia* (eds M. Spitzer *et al*), pp. 70–87. New York: Springer.

WIGGINS, O. P., SCHWARTZ, M. A. & NORTHOFF, G. (1990) Toward a Husserlian phenomenology of the initial stages of schizophrenia. In *Philosophy and Psychopathology* (eds M. Spitzer & B. Maher), pp. 21–34. New York: Springer.

12 Thought insertion, insight and Descartes' *cogito*: linguistic analysis and the descriptive psychopathology of schizophrenic thought disorder

K. W. M. FULFORD

Descartes' *cogito* – "cogito ergo sum", "I think therefore I am" – is among the most famous of philosophical aphorisms. It is also among the most widely criticised. Its first publication (other than in the original Latin) was in conjunction with a series of articles contesting Descartes' arguments together with his replies (an early example of peer review publication); and since Descartes' time philosophers have conceived a wide range of objections to the *cogito* (Williams, 1978).

The schizophrenic symptom of thought insertion appears to contradict the *cogito*. To the extent that thought insertion involves thinking *other* people's thoughts, it seems to amount to an empirical counterexample to the claim that '*I* am' follows from '*I* think'. Thought insertion should thus be of interest to philosophers. Correspondingly, the philosophical literature analysing the *cogito* should be of interest to psychopathologists. Despite its clinical significance, the loss of insight by which thought insertion and related schizophrenic symptoms are characterised is not well understood. Yet until recently, thought insertion has been ignored even by the growing number of philosophers interested in psychopathology; and conversely, even philosophically minded psychopathologists (including Jaspers, 1913, 1965) have ignored the *cogito*.

This chapter brings the two sides together. A brief description is given of Descartes' *cogito* and of the prima facie philosophical significance of thought insertion. This will suggest that one reason why philosophers have neglected thought insertion is because psychopathologists have not recognised just how odd a symptom thought insertion really is. An account of thought insertion is then outlined which draws on the results of work in the philosophy of mind. An adequate differential diagnosis of thought insertion, in particular of the specifically psychotic loss of insight which it involves, is shown to imply a model of rationality in which the affective and intentional aspects of thought and behaviour are as important as the cognitive. This then leads to a reconsideration of the *cogito* and to the conclusion that within this enlarged picture of rationality, Descartes' position, far from being undermined by thought insertion, is actually endorsed by it.

Descartes' cogito and thought insertion

The *cogito* was the pivotal step in the search by the 17th-century rationalist philosopher René Descartes for a secure foundation for knowledge (Descartes, 1968). His approach to this problem has become known as the method of doubt. Instead of looking for something indubitable from which to start, Descartes began by doubting everything that can possibly be doubted. He noted that appearances can be deceptive, that even his own body might be a figment of his imagination, his whole life a delusion. This was suggested empirically by everyday experiences such as error and dreaming. In principle there could be an 'evil demon' with infinite powers who was capable of deceiving us in any and all respects. And yet, Descartes continued, so long as I try to think that everything is false, there is one thing that *is* indubitable, namely that I think. However ingenious the evil demon may be in making me think this or that particular false thought, it is still necessary that I think in order for me to have a thought which is false. As Ayer (1976) put it, "I cannot be mistaken in believing that I exist, since my denial or even my doubt of my own existence itself implies it".

The substance of the *cogito* was anticipated by St Augustine. Moreover, much that Descartes tried to build on the *cogito* is considerably less secure than he claimed – in this sense the *cogito* fails as a foundation. Nonetheless, the *cogito* itself, as already noted, has sustained continuous philosophical interest since its first publication. Its intuitive force arises from what the philosopher Gilbert Ryle (1949) called the 'adhesiveness' of experience, that is, the way in which our experiences are stuck apparently indissolubly to our sense of ourselves as subjects. I can imagine myself without an arm, say, perhaps even without a body. In this sense I can detach my sense of myself as a subject from my body. But my experience, as Ryle put it, is as "inescapable as a shadow".

This adhesiveness is a feature not just of thoughts but of any conscious experience. It is illustrated in Fig. 12.1 for the case of headache. So natural is the adhesiveness between the self and conscious experience that we take it for granted. If I have a headache the last thing I am concerned about is whether it is *my* headache. Such a question, we might feel, could only occur to a philosopher. And yet it is just this separation of the self from experience that we find in the case of thought insertion.

Consider one of Mellor's case histories (Mellor, 1970). The patient, a 29-year-old housewife says:

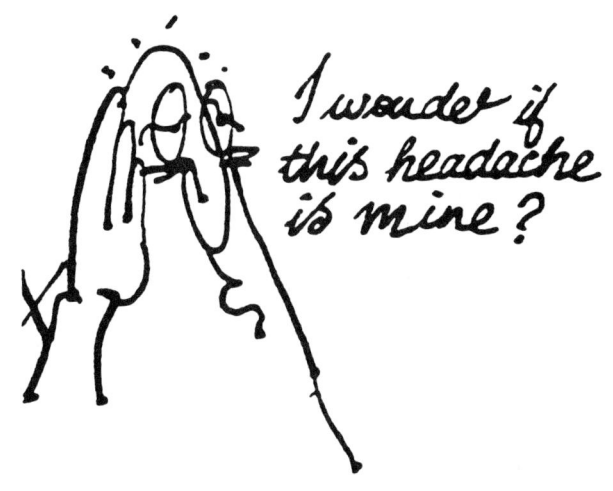

Fig. 12.1. *The adhesiveness of experience. It is easy to imagine losing an arm or an eye; it is not too difficult to imagine being separated from one's whole body; but our conscious experiences seem indissolubly connected with our sense of self. This "adhesiveness of experience" (Ryle, 1949) has been assumed by most philosophers, including Descartes. It is contradicted by thought insertion*

> "I look out of the window and I think the garden looks nice and the grass looks cool. But the thoughts of Eamonn Andrews come into my mind. There are no other thoughts there, only his. He treats my mind like a screen and flashes his thoughts on to it like you flash a picture."

Here then is an experience which appears directly to contradict the *cogito*. The patient, it seems, has a thought in her own head. In this sense, *she* is thinking it. But she experiences it as the thought *of someone else*, of Eamonn Andrews. The normal adhesion between the self and experience is thus broken. Instead of "I think, therefore I am", we have "I think, therefore Eamonn Andrews is," or, more generally, "I think therefore *you* are", "cogito ergo *es*".

Yet thought insertion has been ignored by philosophers. Why? It is certainly not for lack of interest. As noted earlier, right from the start, the *cogito* has been the subject of intense and usually critical philosophical scrutiny. Nor is it for lack of interest in psychopathology, at any rate recently. As Quinton (1985) remarked, it is true that philosophers, in a sense the experts on rationality, have been remarkably slow to show an interest in *ir*rationality. This has now started to change. Philosophical attention has thus far been focused mainly on more immediately arresting (although sometimes dubious) entities such as multiple personality disorder (Gillett, 1986; Braude, 1991). I have argued elsewhere that this is because the more philosophically significant areas of psychopathology, such as evaluative delusions, are not so readily accessible to philosophers (Fulford, 1991a). But the philosophical relevance of thought insertion is transparent.

The question thus remains, why has thought insertion been neglected by philosophers? In the next section it is argued that one reason is that psychiatrists themselves have not taken the oddity of thought insertion seriously enough.

Thought insertion and insight

At first glance it might seem wrong to suggest that psychiatrists have underestimated the oddity of thought insertion. After all, in any standard text it is emphasised that the diagnosis of thought insertion depends on just this, on recognising that it is a lot odder than a range of other experiences – normal and pathological – with which it might be confused. The point is generally made negatively, that is, by contrasting thought insertion with these other experiences. Thus thought insertion is *not* the experience of one's own thoughts being influenced by others, whether by ordinary persuasion or by telepathy or other delusional means (Wing *et al*, 1974). Similarly, it is *not* the experience of one's thoughts being 'out of control'. All thinking, like movement, is partly automatic – our thoughts just run on. In obsessional disorders the loss of control may be so extreme and the content of the obsessions so unpleasant (involving, say, violent or sexual imagery) that patients may describe their thoughts as not their own. As Sims (1988) emphasises, however, this is not to claim, as the patient with thought insertion claims, that their thoughts are really those of anyone else. It is rather to distance oneself from them; it is to say "I am not really *like* that!", "that's not *me*!".

So at one level – at the level of everyday experience – we are well aware that thought insertion is odd. This is connected with the philosophical emphasis on the adhesiveness between our sense of self and our conscious experience noted earlier. This notion, indeed, derived as it is from the philosophy of mind rather than descriptive psychopathology, gives us a positive way of characterising the symptom. Thought insertion is odd just in that the adhesion between the self and experience fails. Most symptoms, mental and physical, differ only in intensity and duration from normal experiences. An obsessional symptom is different only in intensity and duration from such experiences as getting a tune stuck in your head. With most symptoms, then, as with all normal experiences, the adhesion between the self and experience holds fast. But with thought insertion, and other related forms of schizophrenic thought disorder, it fails.

However – and we come now to insight – thought insertion is odder even than this. The point can be made directly in terms of differential diagnosis. As an experience, thought insertion, odd though it is, is not unique. As Lishman (1978) describes, 'forced' thoughts may occur in the aura of temporal lobe epilepsy, and this may be similar to thought insertion. Thought insertion, it is true, is generally more persistent and less stereotyped. The key difference, though, is that with temporal lobe epilepsy patients more or less readily accept that their forced thoughts, rather than being those of some other agency, are, straightforwardly, a symptom of something wrong with them. It is this insight which the patient with true thought insertion lacks. And it is this which shows that thought insertion is odder than has generally been appreciated because, essentially, this specifically psychotic loss of insight is itself odder than has generally been appreciated.

The standard account of insight stems from Aubrey Lewis's paper "On the psychopathology of insight", published in 1934. This paper sets a high standard for philosophical psychopathology. The line of argument is developed with great clarity and it is richly illustrated with vivid clinical examples. Aubrey Lewis came out against insight, however. He argued that, so far at least as insight is the basis of the traditional distinction between psychotic and non-psychotic disorders, it lacks empirical content and has no place in a properly scientific psychopathology. Thus he defined insight as a "correct attitude to a morbid change in oneself". This definition, as he noted, requires some elaboration, but however carefully this is carried out, clinical experience shows that there are patients with (traditionally) non-psychotic disorders (and indeed patients with physical disorders) who lack insight, so defined, and similarly that there are patients with (traditionally) psychotic disorders whose insight is well preserved. Hence, he concluded, the psychotic/non-psychotic distinction should be abandoned.

This has become the official line. In ICD-9, for instance, the psychotic/non-psychotic distinction was retained, although somewhat grudgingly (World Health Organization, 1978). In ICD-10 (World Health Organization, 1992), following DSM-III (American Psychiatric Association, 1980), it has ostensibly been dropped. The difficulty, though, for the official line, is that, unlike a number of other psychopathological distinctions (e.g. endogenous versus reactive depression), the psychotic/non-psychotic distinction persists. It persists in everyday psychiatric usage and in academic journals, in expressions like antipsychotic drug and puerperal psychosis; it persists in the continuing significance of psychotic disorders in medicolegal and ethical contexts, such as involuntary psychiatric treatment (Fulford, 1991*b*); and, more remarkably, it persists even in our official classifications. DSM and ICD both have subcategories of psychotic disorders, and even a category for "psychotic disorders not elsewhere classified" (DSM section II; ICD F28). Indeed, appearances notwithstanding, the place of the psychotic/non-psychotic distinction in DSM-III and ICD-10 can be shown to be strictly equivalent to its place in ICD-9 (Fulford, 1994).

The persistence of a concept in this way is open to a number of interpretations. It could be a reflection of inertia, say. However, a more positive interpretation is suggested by the work of the Oxford philosopher J. L. Austin, and others, sometimes called 'ordinary language philosophy' or 'linguistic analysis' (Austin, 1956–57; Fulford, 1989*b*). Linguistic analysis is based on the observation that we are often better at using concepts than at defining them: standard philosophical examples of this include the concepts of time and baroque. According to this approach, the persistent *use* of a concept, despite difficulties of definition, suggests that the concept in question is serving an important function in our language (Fulford, 1989a, Ch. 10). In other words, it is helping us to say something that we need to say. In psychiatry we tend to assume that the effective use of a concept depends on the availability of a clear, explicit definition. This is sometimes true – the concept of schizophrenia has been put to better use as a result of clearer definition (Cooper *et al*, 1972). But the persistence of the psychotic/non-psychotic distinction *despite* evident difficulties of definition suggests, rather, that Aubrey Lewis's failure to differentiate psychotic from non-psychotic disorders could be a failure, not of the concept of psychotic loss of insight, but of his proposed definition. Instead of abandoning the psychotic/non-psychotic distinction, then, what is needed is better understanding of psychotic loss of insight.

Philosophy of mind and insight

After a period of relative neglect there has been something of a revival of interest in the psychopathology of insight. This has involved a variety of disciplines, including psychiatry, psychology, anthropology, and, not least, philosophy (Amador & David, 1994). Many of these approaches can be understood as involving a return to the traditional medical emphasis on the importance of careful attention to the patient's actual experiences. As we have seen, this is also central to the method of linguistic analysis in philosophy. Linguistic analysis, moreover, incorporates a particular view of the likely nature of difficulties of definition, namely that they often arise from a tendency to take too narrow or restricted a view of the meanings of the concepts in question (Fulford, 1989b). Hence exploring the ways in which these concepts are actually used can help to give us a more complete understanding of their meanings.

Applying this to psychotic loss of insight suggests that the difficulties encountered by Aubrey Lewis and his successors may indeed have arisen from taking too narrow a view of the meanings of psychopathological concepts. Aubrey Lewis worked within what has become known as the 'medical' model. According to this model, the concepts of illness and disease, including therefore all psychopathological concepts, are essentially factual concepts. They involve disturbances of functioning on which doctors, as scientists, are experts. This model is evident in the language in which Aubrey Lewis develops his account (Lewis, 1934). Thus a correct "attitude" turns out to be one which is all to do with "data" and "observation of change"; and a "correct" attitude "approximates to that of the physician". Moreover, a "morbid change", he says, is a disturbance of "part-functioning", thus anticipating an explicitly medical model of the meaning of disease which he developed in detail in a later paper (Lewis, 1955).

There is nothing wrong with the scientific medical model as such. On the contrary, it reflects the success of science in medicine generally, and the empirical approach continues to be important in work on insight, as in the studies reported by David (1990), for instance. Moreover, it can be shown to be sufficient to encompass some forms of loss of insight. This is especially so with the cognitive symptoms associated with organic psychoses – global cognitive loss in dementia, for instance, and visual neglect after certain forms of stroke (Fulford, 1993a). But the patient's actual experience in the case of thought insertion is quite different from these. With organic psychotic loss of insight there is merely a passive lack of awareness of incapacity. The patient is simply not aware that there is anything wrong. In the case of non-organic, or so-called functional, psychotic loss of insight, on the other hand, what is wrong is *actively* relocated by the patient as something that is being done *to* them by someone else.

This way of contrasting organic and functional psychotic losses of insight is capable of generating complex differential diagnostic tables for a wide variety of psychotic symptoms (Fulford, 1989a, Ch. 10). A table for thought insertion is illustrated in Table 12.1. Here, thought insertion is distinguished from normal thoughts, obsessional thoughts and epileptic 'forced' thoughts. Normal thoughts are things we do, albeit often more or less automatically, and often to a greater or lesser extent influenced by others. Hence, when we

TABLE 12.1
A differential illness – diagnosis of thought insertion

Conscious experience	Construal					
	By patient			By others		
	Done by	Wrong with	Done to	Done by	Wrong with	Done to
Normal thoughts	+			+		
Thoughts influenced by others	+			+		
Obsessional thoughts		+			+	
Epileptic 'forced' thoughts		+			+	
Another person's thoughts (*thought insertion*)			+		+	

This table compares the patient's understanding of a variety of 'thought experiences' with the way in which they are understood by others, across a two-way distinction by which the subjective experience of illness is (partly) defined. The experience of illness, mental and bodily, is distinct both from the experience of things being done *to* us and from that of *doing* things (Fulford, 1989a, Ch. 7). This two-way distinction, as an important general feature of the experience of illness, is also the starting point for an account of insight which, in contrast to traditional accounts, is capable of differentiating functional psychotic from non-psychotic symptoms. This is illustrated in the table by the way in which thought insertion stands out from other thought experiences. With normal thoughts, thoughts influenced by others, obsessional thoughts, and even epileptic 'forced' thoughts (once their nature is explained to the patient), there is congruence between the patient's experience and the construction placed on that experience by others (represented respectively by the two halves of the table). It is only with thought insertion that there is a mismatch.

really do lose control of our thoughts, the experience is of something wrong. With obsessional and epileptic thoughts, for instance, there is loss of control, and with both these non-psychotic symptoms the experience is construed by the patient and by everyone else as something wrong. For symptoms such as these, there is congruence between the patient and everyone else. But with thought insertion, and only with thought insertion, this congruence breaks down. Here everyone else construes the experience as something wrong while the patient construes it as something that is done *to* them. From the perspective of the patient in Mellor's paper, for example, Eamonn Andrews was using her mind, moving her thoughts, doing something *to* her, rather as he might move her arm.

I have elsewhere called tables of this kind differential illness–diagnostic tables to emphasise the fact that they are constructed directly in terms of the patient's actual experience of illness rather than indirectly in terms of medical knowledge of disease (Fulford, 1993*a*). The patient's experience, broadly, is of incapacity, of being unable to do things that one can ordinarily do. This is represented in the table (for the case of thinking) by a shift from the left-hand column to the centre column, a shift from the experience of 'doing something' to the experience of 'something wrong with me'. With other symptoms the right-hand column is also important: paralysis, for example, as something wrong with me, is different both from being restrained (something done to me) and from simply not moving (something I do). But a table along these lines can in principle be constructed for any experience of illness, physical or mental, non-psychotic or psychotic (Fulford, 1989*a*, Ch. 10).

Differential illness–diagnostic tables, therefore, elementary as the approach may seem, represent a potentially powerful heuristic device. What is implied by such tables, though, is that if we are to gain a better understanding of the psychopathology of insight, and hence of symptoms like thought insertion, we must be prepared to entertain and work with a range of concepts more familiar in the philosophy of mind than in (medical) science. For *doing* things, although contingently dependent on the integrity of the functional systems emphasised by the scientific medical model, is a property of *agents*: arms and legs, for example, livers and lungs, all function; but agents (paradigmatically, people like you and me) perform *actions*. It is a failure of action which is the essence of the experience of incapacity and hence of illness (Fulford, 1989*a*, Ch. 7); and the analysis of actions involves motives, intentions, subjectivity, values, free will, rationality, and other concepts with which philosophers, rather than scientists, have traditionally been concerned.

It is from a philosophical psychopathology, therefore, not replacing but complementing the traditional descriptive psychopathology, that we should expect better understanding of the experience of illness, and hence of insight, to emerge. There are clear indications of this in some of the recent work on insight. Perkins & Moodley (1993), for example, have noted the cultural relativity of standards of insight, and Markova & Berrios (1992) have pointed to the importance of the affective and evaluative aspects of belief formation. Linguistic analysis helps to show this directly in terms of the conceptual framework required for an adequate differential diagnosis of the symptoms themselves.

Psychopathology and the philosophy of mind

The approach outlined here is not anti-scientific. Rather, it shows science and philosophy as twin resources for the development of clinical psychopathology.

Ryle's concept of the adhesiveness of experience provides a positive way of characterising what is so odd about thought insertion, complementing the standard accounts in which it is explained mainly by contrasting it with other symptoms. Deeper understanding of thought insertion, and hence of the loss of insight by which psychotic symptoms as a whole are characterised, will depend, if the ideas outlined here are correct, on deeper understanding of the nature of intentional action. I have taken this argument further elsewhere (Fulford, 1989a). Work in this area has, thus far, been carried out mainly by philosophers. Searle's work, in particular, on the structure of intentionality, provides a rich framework of ideas for exploring the psychopathology of delusion (Fulford, 1993b). If we are to make progress in understanding our key psychopathological concepts, it is likely that we will find ourselves drawn into areas which are as much philosophical as scientific.

If philosophy is a resource for psychopathology, the converse is also true. This indeed may be an area in which, as Austin (1956–57) put it, it is the negative concept which wears the trousers. What Austin had in mind was that we can often gain important insights into the meanings of our concepts by looking at situations in which things go wrong – a conceptual counterpart to diabetes leading to the discovery of insulin (Fulford, 1989b). Where everything works smoothly we are, as he said, blinded by "ease and obviousness". Hence if we are interested in the nature of action, we should look not to normal actions but to situations in which actions fail. Austin himself drew on court reports as a philosophical database of excuses (these involving various kinds of failure of action); but at the end of his paper, perhaps anticipating the development of philosophical psychopathology, he pointed to abnormal psychological phenomena as an even richer resource for work in this area.

Austin's point is well illustrated by the significance of thought insertion (and related symptoms) for the philosophy of mind. For rather as psychiatrists have underestimated the oddity of thought insertion, so philosophers have underestimated the *cogito*. In particular:

(a) they have failed to recognise that the adhesiveness between the self and experience *can* be broken
(b) their approach has been *too exclusively cognitive*
(c) they have often failed to consider *non*-cognitive approaches.

Thus, on the adhesiveness of experience, there has been much philosophical speculation on the divisibility of persons – subpersonal minds (Minsky, 1987), split brains (Churchland, 1986), even thought experiments involving matter transmitters and brain transplants (Parfit, 1984). Throughout, though, it has been assumed that the self goes with experience – subpersonal persons are generally not attributed experiences at all. But in split-brain experiments the two 'halves' retain their own experiences, and if, as in one of Parfit's (1984) thought experiments, I split into two, the two 'mes' then both say *I* think or *I* have a headache; the two 'mes' both own their thoughts and headaches.

This assumption of adhesiveness is general. It is implicit in the *cogito*, and Descartes elsewhere makes it explicit: writing of himself as a "thinking thing", he says "[I] conceive myself as one single and complete thing" (Descartes, 1968, Sixth Meditation). Here are a few other examples: "'I think' [must] accompany all my representations" (Kant, 1966); experiences cannot "rove about the world" (Frege, 1967); "I . . . always indicates me and only me" (Ryle, 1949); ". . . consciousness is never experienced in the plural, only the singular" (Schrödinger, 1967); there is no room for a ". . . mistake about who is doing the doubting" (Glover, 1988).

By extension, then, thought insertion, undermining as it does the widespread philosophical assumption of adhesiveness, has a widespread significance for the philosophy of mind. It is not just an oddity, moreover. As the philosopher Ruth Chadwick (1994) has shown, it can be a valuable heuristic tool, helping to advance understanding even of such well researched ideas as Kant's treatment of personal identity. Yet as we have seen, philosophers, including Kant, and indeed Descartes himself, have almost always assumed that the self and experience are inseparable.

In much of the philosophical work just noted it has been a cognitive or scientific paradigm which is dominant. There are signs of a shift of approach recently, but even so, the thought experiments still so widely employed in philosophy clearly reflect the influence of this paradigm – split brains, matter transmitters, and so forth. Much the same was true of both Descartes and his opponents. Descartes took the *cogito* to establish the existence of mind as a *substance*, an immaterial substance, to be sure, but a substance none the less. Kant, similarly, an early critic of the *cogito*, argued that it failed to prove the existence of an enduring *object* – the self. Indeed, the whole debate about dualism is full of scientific images – coincident clocks, interaction of mind and brain via the pineal, and so forth. Similarly, David Hume, the 18th-century British empiricist, sought to explore the concept of personal identity by means of (cognitive) introspection (although – shades of Aubrey Lewis here – not finding it, he rejected it; Hume, 1962).

The paradigm of the natural sciences, then, as Wittgenstein was aware (Lee, 1980), has been perhaps too dominant in philosophy. There is an alternative. As with the standard account of psychopathology, the point is not that the cognitive approach is wrong; rather, it is incomplete. On personal identity, for instance, Locke (1960) emphasised the moral or forensic significance of personhood. I am *responsible* in a way a machine is not. This theme has recently been taken up by philosophers such as Harry Frankfurt (1971) and Derek Parfit (1984). What is shown by thought insertion, however, and the psychotic loss of insight by which it is defined, is something stronger even than this. Thought insertion shows, not merely that persons have moral significance, but that the adhesion between the self and experience is, as the philosophers Stephens & Graham (1994) have put it, "agentic" rather than merely cognitive. To own an experience, that is to say, is not just to be directly aware of it. It is to connect it with the motives and intentions by which we are marked out *as* agents.

Finally, what of Descartes himself? Would he have been disconcerted by thought insertion? Well, perhaps at first. As noted earlier, thought insertion is an empirical counterexample to the intuitively persuasive move from 'I think' to 'I am'. However, closer inspection shows, on the contrary, that the *cogito* is reinforced by the separation of 'I' from 'my experience' in thought insertion. Briefly, the point is that although the intuitive force of the *cogito* comes from the adhesiveness of experience, this is also the basis of an important objection to it, pointed out by Kant (1966). Thus, so long as I and my experience can be assumed to be *in*separable, '*I think*' shows only that *thinking* exists, not that *I* exist. Hence Descartes' search for a secure foundation for knowledge, to the extent that it depends on the certainty that 'I exist', fails. However, if, as is shown by thought insertion, my thoughts *can* be separated from my sense of self, if *I* can think *other* people's thoughts, then *I* think really does show that *I* am. There is no endorsement here for the superstructure of theory which Descartes sought to build on the *cogito*. Thought insertion offers no support for mind–body dualism, for instance; nor does it somehow prove the existence of an "enduring ego". Descartes was surely wrong in both these, as it were, cognitive empirical claims. But if 'I' and 'think' can be unstuck, then '*I* think' really does entail '*I* am'.

Conclusions

Thought insertion thus has at least a prima facie relevance to philosophical work on the *cogito* and, indeed, given the pervasiveness of the assumption of adhesiveness, more generally for other questions in the philosophy of mind.

Moreover, the requirements for an adequate clinical account of psychotic loss of insight – the non-cognitive as well as cognitive requirements – correlate closely with the growing philosophical recognition of the importance of the affective, evaluative, and conative elements of rationality. There are clearly some broad themes to be followed through in these areas. Thought insertion illustrates the potential importance of specific kinds of psychopathology, of the details of the phenomena with which psychiatrists are concerned day to day, even for the most abstract of philosophical questions. It may be that philosophy will turn out to have something to contribute to psychopathology. It is certain that psychopathology has much to contribute to philosophy.

Acknowledgements

I am grateful to Professor Ruth Chadwick for her helpful comments on an early draft of this paper and to the Open University for permission to reproduce the cartoon character in Fig. 12.1.

References

AMADOR, X. F. & DAVID, A. S. (1994) *Insight and Psychosis.* Oxford: Oxford University Press (in press).
AMERICAN PSYCHIATRIC ASSOCIATION (1980) *Diagnostic and Statistical Manual of Mental Disorder* (3rd edn) (DSM-III). Washington, DC: APA.
AUSTIN, J. L. (1956–57) A plea for excuses. Proceedings of the Aristotelian Society. Reprinted in *The Philosophy of Action* (ed. A. R. White, 1968). Oxford: Oxford University Press.
AYER, A. J. (1976) *The Central Questions of Philosophy.* Harmondsworth: Penguin.
BRAUDE, S. E. (1991) *First Person Plural: Multiple Personality Disorder and the Philosophy of Mind.* London: Routledge.
CHADWICK, R. (1994) Kant, thought insertions and mental unity. *Philosophy, Psychiatry and Psychology,* **1**, 105–114.
CHURCHLAND, P. (1988) Reduction and the neurobiological basis of consciousness. In *Consciousness in Contemporary Science* (eds A. J. Marcel & E. Bisiach). Oxford: Oxford University Press.
COOPER, J. E., KENDELL, R. E., GURLAND, B. J., *et al* (1972) *Psychiatric Diagnosis in New York and London.* Maudsley Monograph No. 20. Oxford: Oxford University Press.
DAVID, A. S. (1990) Insight and psychosis. *British Journal of Psychiatry,* **156**, 798–808.
DENNET, D. C. (1976) Conditions of personhood. In *Identities of Persons* (ed. O. A. Rorty). Berkeley: University of California Press.
DESCARTES, R. (1968) *Discourse of Method and Meditations* (trans. F. E. Sutcliffe). Harmondsworth: Penguin.
FRANKFURT, H. G. (1971) Freedom of the will and the concept of a person. *Journal of Philosophy,* **68**, 15–20.
FREGE, G. (1967) Thought: A Logical Enquiry (trans. A. Quinton). In *Philosophical Logic* (ed. P. F. Strawson). Oxford: Oxford University Press.
FULFORD, K. W. M. (1989a) *Moral Theory and Medical Practice.* Cambridge: Cambridge University Press.
––––– (1989b) Philosophy and medicine: the Oxford connection. *British Journal of Psychiatry,* **157**, 111–115.
––––– (1991a) Evaluative delusions: their significance for philosophy and psychiatry. *British Journal of Psychiatry,* **159**, (suppl. 14), 108–112.

—— (1991*b*) The concept of disease. In *Psychiatric Ethics* (2nd edn) (eds S. Bloch & P. Chodoff). Oxford: Oxford University Press.

—— (1993*a*) Thought insertion and insight: disease and illness paradigms of psychotic disorder. In *Phenomenology, Language and Schizophrenia* (ed. M. Spitzer). New York: Springer-Verlag.

—— (1993*b*) Mental illness and mind–brain problem: delusion, belief and Searle's theory of intentionality. *Theoretical Medicine*, **14**, 181–194.

—— (1994) Closet logics: hidden conceptual elements in the DSM and ICD classifications of mental disorders. In *Philosophical Perspectives on Psychiatric Diagnostic Classification* (eds J. Z. Sadler, M. Schwartz & O. Wiggins). Baltimore: Johns Hopkins University Press.

GILLETT, G. R. (1986) Multiple personality and the concept of a person. *New Ideas in Psychology*, **4**, 173–184.

GLOVER, J. (1988) *I: The Philosophy and Psychology of Personal Identity*. London: Penguin.

HUME, D. (1962) Of personal identity. Book I, Part IV, Section IV. In *A Treatise of Human Nature* (ed. D. G. C. Macnabb). Glasgow: Fontana/Collins.

JASPERS, K. (1913) *General Psychopathology* (trans. J. Hoenig & M. W. Hamilton, 1963). Manchester: Manchester University Press.

—— (1965) Descartes and philosophy. In *Leonardo, Descartes, Max Weber: Three Essays* (trans. R. Manheim). London: Routledge & Kegan Paul.

KANT, I. (1966) *The Critique of Pure Reason* (trans. N. Kemp Smith). New York: Doubleday.

LEE, D. (ed.) *Wittgenstein's Lectures: Cambridge, 1930–1932*. Oxford: Blackwell.

LEWIS, A. J. (1934) On the psychopathology of insight. *British Journal of Medicine and Psychology*, **14**, 332–348.

—— (1955) Health as a social concept. *British Journal of Sociology*, **4**, 109–124.

LISHMAN, A. W. (1978) *Organic Psychiatry*. Oxford: Blackwell Scientific.

LOCKE, J. (1960) Of identity and diversity. Essays, Book II, Ch. xxvii. In *John Locke: An Essay Concerning Human Understanding* (ed. A. D. Woozley). London: Fontana.

MARKOVA, I. S. & BERRIOS, G. E. (1992) The meaning of insight in clinical psychiatry. *British Journal of Psychiatry*, **160**, 850–860.

MELLOR, C. S. (1970) First rank symptoms of schizophrenia. *British Journal of Psychiatry*, **117**, 15–23.

MINSKY, M. (1987) *The Society of Mind*. Great Britain: Heinemann.

PARFIT, D. (1984) *Reasons and Persons*. Oxford: Clarendon Press.

PERKINS, R. & MOODLEY, P. (1993) The arrogance of insight. *Psychiatric Bulletin*, **17**, 233–234.

QUINTON, A. (1955) Madness. In *Philosophy and Practice* (ed. A. P. Griffiths). Cambridge: Cambridge University Press.

RYLE, G. (1949) *The Concept of Mind*. London: Hutchinson.

SCHRÖDINGER, E. (1967) *Mind and Matter*. Cambridge: Cambridge University Press.

SIMS, A. (1988) *Symptoms in the Mind: A Introduction to Descriptive Psychopathology*. London: Baillière Tindall.

STEPHENS, G. L. & GRAHAM, G. (1994) Self-consciousness, mental agency and the clinical psychopathology. *Philosophy, Psychiatry and Psychology*, **1**, 1–10.

WILLIAMS, B. (1978) *Descartes: The Project of Pure Enquiry*. Harmondsworth: Penguin.

WING, J. K., COOPER, J. E. & SARTORIUS, N. (1974) *Measurement and Classification of Psychiatric Symptoms*. Cambridge: Cambridge University Press.

WORLD HEALTH ORGANIZATION (1978) *Mental Disorders: Glossary and Guide to Their Classification in Accordance with the Ninth Revision of the International Classification of Diseases* (ICD-9). Geneva: WHO.

—— (1992) *The ICD-10 Classification of Mental and Behavioural Disorders: Clinical Descriptions and Diagnostic Guidelines*. Geneva: WHO.

Part III. Other psychiatric disorders

13 Some aspects of language disorder in dementia

EDGAR MILLER

Anyone who has worked with people who have dementia is aware that language becomes impaired. Speech is impoverished, there can be difficulties in word finding or naming, and so on. That language impairments occur is not in serious dispute; indeed, it would be remarkable if a degenerative disease of the nervous system which has such a wide impact on the brain and psychological functioning were to leave language totally spared.

The key question is, therefore, not whether language impairments exist in dementia, but what is their nature? Also, how do language disturbances relate to other impairments and, eventually, what if anything might be done to ameliorate the handicapping effects of deteriorating language? This chapter explores these issues with respect to dementia of the Alzheimer type. It is possible that language is affected in different ways in the different types of dementia. Given the constraints of space and the available information, this chapter concentrates on the one type of dementia, and further use of the term 'dementia', unless otherwise qualified, is intended to refer solely to dementia of the Alzheimer type.

Methodological problems

Before looking at the evidence, it is sensible to take note of some of the limitations that arise in studying language ability in people with dementia. Several major problems can be identified.

Firstly, the fact that so many different aspects of functioning are adversely affected in dementia can make it difficult to discriminate failures in performance due to language deficits from failures due to other kinds of deficits: is a failure to name an object or picture of an object due to a real inability to name as opposed to a perceptual difficulty in identifying the objects to be named?

Secondly, while theoretical models of language do exist, and in abundance, these have not been widely exploited in looking at language in dementia. In a highly complex area it is useful to have some guiding theoretical principle to follow, if only on a heuristic basis, and this has generally been lacking. Much of the work so far has been centred on particular language-related tasks, and has been relatively atheoretical.

Thirdly, dementia is a steadily progressive disorder. This means that any full analysis of language in dementia needs to look at how language problems begin and then develop. This implies the use of longitudinal studies or at least cross-sectional studies which look at groups of subjects with differing lengths of illness. With a few exceptions, this sort of work has not yet been carried out.

Fourthly, there is the problem of defining the populations to be studied. The identification of Alzheimer-type dementia is not an exact science, especially in the early stages, and it is sometimes difficult to determine exactly what diagnostic criteria were used in much of the reported work.

Finally, language can be affected by sensory handicaps, especially deafness, and sensory handicaps are common in the age range of concern in studying dementia. Again, published reports typically do not say much about the sensory assessment of the subjects being studied, and the reader is left to assume that sensory impairments were not a crucial factor. It may well be that such assumptions are not always valid.

Nature of language impairment

The literature on language impairment in Alzheimer-type dementia is now quite large. Some key points and examples are discussed below; more detailed reviews are given by Miller (1989) and Miller & Morris (1993).

Before looking at the effect of dementia on different types of language-related tasks, a preliminary point needs to be mentioned. It has been claimed that certain subgroups of people suffering from Alzheimer-type dementia are more likely to develop language impairments than others. In particular, it has been suggested that those with an earlier onset, a more rapid progression of the disorder, and stronger evidence of a genetic transmission are more likely to have language problems. Evidence consistent with this view has been reported by Breitner & Folstein (1984), Faber-Langendoen et al (1988) and Seltzer & Sherwin (1983). While this might be a commonly reported picture it is certainly not found in all relevant studies. For example, Bayles (1991) has reported that certain types of language impairment might be more prevalent in those with an older age of onset. A possible cause of confusion with regard to the evidence linking language impairments to age of onset is that age of onset is only one potentially relevant factor. Other potentially relevant factors, like length of illness, need to be taken into account before firm conclusions can be reached, and these have generally not been properly controlled for.

Aphasia and language impairment in dementia

One approach to language in dementia has been to draw on work on aphasia. A number of investigations have used instruments or batteries of tests designed to identify subtypes of aphasia (e.g. Appell *et al*, 1982; Cummings *et al*, 1985). The underlying assumption appears to be that language impairment in dementia is a form of aphasia due to focal lesions of the brain. The results of these studies have often been considered to indicate that dementia produces one subtype of aphasia or another. The problem is that if batteries of language tests are applied of a kind specifically designed to detect different subtypes of aphasia, then any subjects with language impairment run the risk of being forced into one category or another of aphasic disorder, regardless.

An early study by Ernst *et al* (1970) found no clear pattern of language impairment but noted poverty of vocabulary and difficulties in naming. On the other hand, both Cummings *et al* (1985) and Murdoch *et al* (1987) reported patterns of language impairment resembling transcortical sensory aphasia.

A research group associated with Kertesz (Appell *et al*, 1982; Kertesz *et al*, 1986) reported more varied patterns of language disorder. Patterns corresponding to transcortical sensory, Wernicke's and global aphasia were claimed. This group has also examined the progression of language impairment by looking at the patterns exhibited by subjects who had been suffering dementia for different lengths of time. They concluded that the language impairment starts with anomic aphasia and passes through transcortical sensory and Wernicke's aphasia before ending up as global aphasia. While it is reasonable to expect that language impairment in dementia is likely to be progressive, it should be noted that this latter conclusion is based on a total of only 25 subjects in a cross-sectional study. No longitudinal studies appear to have been conducted.

Finally, an investigation by Bayles (1982) should be mentioned. A large number of tests, many of which are similar to those used in aphasia assessments, were administered to elderly patients with dementia and controls. Poor language functioning was found in the group with dementia, and Bayles reported that the semantic aspects of language were more liable to disruption than the phonological or syntactic. This is reasonably consistent with the research based on aphasia batteries in suggesting a predominance of impairments akin to the more posteriorly linked forms of aphasia.

Work in this tradition does appear to suggest that language impairments in dementia more or less map onto patterns of aphasia associated with focal lesions of the left hemisphere and especially the more posterior forms of aphasia, such as transcortical sensory and Wernicke's aphasia. However, as has already been indicated, the methods adopted are likely to push any demonstrated language deficits into patterns found in focal aphasia. There are other investigations of language based on different types of measure which appear to show differences in the nature of the language impairment between those with dementia and those with aphasia due to focal lesions (e.g. Rochford, 1971; Code & Lodge, 1987; Margolin *et al*, 1990). These studies are not described here, but are taken up later in their appropriate context.

Naming

The specific language function that appears to have attracted most attention in relation to dementia is naming, and there is no doubt that patients with this disorder do have an impaired ability to name things (e.g. Barker & Lawson, 1968; Lawson & Barker, 1968). Early on, Stengel (1964) suggested that the naming errors of demented subjects differed from those associated with aphasia due to focal lesions, in that aphasic subjects give the impression of knowing the object to be named but being unable to supply the name. In contrast, demented subjects appear not to appreciate what the object is, and to supply a name for an object that they misperceive. Additional support for this notion came from studies reported by Rochford (1971).

That those with dementia may have perceptual impairments and that perceptual difficulties might lead to misnaming is far from implausible. Indeed, other studies have shown that degraded and more difficult to perceive pictures of objects have a much more deleterious effect on naming in dementia than in other disorders (Kirschner *et al*, 1984), as would be expected if perceptual impairments were at least partly responsible. It therefore seems to be the case that, under some conditions at least, errors in naming are caused by faulty perception.

The key question, then, is whether all naming problems can be explained in this way. Again, the answer is fairly unequivocal and points to situations where truly linguistic factors are involved. For example, Huff *et al* (1986) screened demented subjects using a test of perceptual discrimination and found that even those who performed entirely normally were still impaired on naming. Similarly, Skelton-Robinson & Jones (1984) prompted subjects on a naming task by supplying definitions of the names that they had failed to provide. This did not enhance naming as might have been expected if naming failures were solely due to misperception.

What seems to have been shown so far is that while misperception of the object or picture to be named can underlie difficulties in naming, at least to some degree, misperception cannot explain all of the impairment. There is at least one additional linguistic component. The next question concerns the nature of that component.

Both Bayles & Tomoeda (1983) and Martin & Fedio (1983) have analysed the errors in naming made by subjects with dementia and concluded that there are semantic difficulties. On the other hand, Bowles *et al* (1987) described naming errors as reflecting difficulties in concept identification and in selecting between possible responses. The problem in analysing errors, as Huff *et al* (1986) pointed out, is that they can be ambiguous and difficult to assign to categories. For example, if the subject is shown a picture of a donkey and responds 'horse', does this reflect a perceptual error (a correct name assigned to a misperceived object), or is this a semantic error (misnaming a correctly perceived object)?

Other types of investigation also suggest a strong semantic component. In a complex experiment designed to examine components of the naming process, Flicker *et al* (1987) claimed that the language impairment in dementia is secondary to problems in semantic memory. Similar conclusions were drawn by Margolin *et al* (1990), who studied both naming and a controlled word association in subjects with dementia as well as subjects with aphasia due to focal lesions. There was a double dissociation, with the demented group being even worse in naming than the aphasic subjects but with the aphasic subjects being worse on the word association test. Apart from clearly demonstrating a difference between aphasia and the language impairment of dementia, these results were claimed as showing that impaired word finding reflects a reduced ability to process semantic information in those with dementia, but undue difficulties with lexical/phonological information in the aphasic group.

This latter pattern of difficulties with the semantic aspects of language in dementia, with relative preservation of the lexical, phonological and indeed the syntactic aspects, does appear quite frequently from work using a variety of language tasks. On the other hand, there are instances where semantic processing seems to be preserved. One example of this is a study of semantic priming by Nebes *et al* (1986). It has been found in research with normal subjects that the speed of naming of a visually presented word (e.g. 'doctor') is enhanced if it is immediately preceded by a semantically related word (e.g. 'nurse'). This effect is known as semantic priming, and Nebes *et al* showed that this effect was as marked in subjects with dementia as in age-matched controls. This implies that whatever semantic features were being tapped by this task had remained reasonably intact.

Negative priming can also be demonstrated in normal subjects, where the appearance of the first word actually retards the second response (e.g. 'nurse–baker' as opposed to 'nurse–doctor'). Hartman (1991) confirmed normal degrees of positive priming in subjects with dementia but failed to show any negative priming in contexts where this appears in normal subjects. This could reflect some semantic peculiarities in dementia, although Hartman opts for a different (inherently less plausible) explanation in terms of alleged differing attention demands of positive and negative priming.

The evidence on naming is far from being wholly consistent. On balance it supports the view that no single mechanism can explain all naming failures under all circumstances. In some contexts, at least, misperception probably plays a role. Nevertheless, there do appear to be true linguistic difficulties underlying the inadequacies in naming, with the strongest indications pointing in the direction of the semantic aspects of language rather than the lexical or phonological.

Conversational speech

Naming tasks are artificial, so it might be useful to consider the production of speech under more natural circumstances like conversation or related situations. Miller & Hague (1975) analysed audiotaped samples of normal conversational speech, and looked at the statistical characteristics of the words used. It might be that demented subjects rely on a smaller range of words than controls; these words would then be used more frequently within samples of similar total word length. No such tendency was found. This implies that the total number of words in the lexicon remains intact, or nearly intact, at least in relatively early cases. Miller & Hague combined this finding with that of a reduced number of words produced in a word fluency task (reported in the same paper). They then concluded that, while the size of the lexicon may be more or less normal, access to the words in the lexicon was either impaired or much slower, but to an equal degree across all words regardless of the frequency with which they are used in everyday speech.

Other investigators have also carried out analyses based upon ordinary conversations or oral descriptions of a picture. Various differences between the speech of demented and normal subjects have been claimed. For example, Hier et al (1985) found that subjects with dementia used fewer words, propositional phrases and subordinate clauses in speech, as well as producing more incomplete sentences. They suggested that lexical defects occurred more frequently than syntactical defects and that problems in accessing the lexicon increased with the severity of the dementia. Comparable findings were reported by Kempler et al (1987) and Nicholas et al (1985).

Hutchinson & Jensen (1980) analysed their conversational material in rather different ways. Their elderly subjects with dementia were like control subjects in that most utterances were statements of belief or assertions. The group with dementia differed in producing a higher rate of directives (questions or requests which require the listener to do something). Rather surprisingly, they also initiated more topics in conversation, but these were largely as a part of what were considered to be violations of the ordinary rules of conversation. Hutchinson & Jensen did not elaborate on this much, but it appears that many of the newly initiated topics introduced by the group with dementia may well have consisted of the introduction of irrelevances into the conversation. In turn, these might be linked to memory impairments resulting in the person losing track of the conversation or in misunderstanding what the interviewer had just said.

In general, conversational speech appears to be impoverished, less elaborate, and more fragmented. A number of investigators have also drawn attention to what appear to be lexical access difficulties in the course of conversational speech.

Comprehension

One of the best methods of testing language comprehension is to use De Renzi & Vignolo's (1962) token test or one of its later versions. Two separate studies (Thompson, 1987; Faber-Langendoen et al, 1988) have shown that subjects with dementia are clearly impaired on the token test. While the token test may work well with aphasic subjects who have focal lesions, it is likely that, under more extreme circumstances, lowered general intellectual functioning or impaired memory could also adversely affect performance. Subjects with dementia show both these features and so these results have to be treated with caution.

Impairments in reading comprehension have also been claimed. One study (Cummings et al, 1986) started by showing that subjects with dementia could read words even when these were obscured by superimposed diagonal lines. This implied that an apparent difficulty in the comprehension of written material could not be ascribed to problems in perception. It was noted that comprehension did appear to be adversely affected in that subjects with dementia could read out written commands that they were unable to perform.

Other investigators have also confirmed that impairments in reading comprehension arise (e.g. Thompson, 1987; Faber-Langendoen et al, 1988). In one study, Schwartz et al (1979) examined a single subject with dementia as well as three with Broca's aphasia. The aphasic subjects appeared to have difficulty with the syntactic aspects of the written communications, while the demented subject had lexical difficulties in the face of a preserved understanding of syntax.

Another study (Kempler et al, 1988) tested the comprehension of single words, familiar phrases, idioms and proverbs, and novel phrases. Those with probable Alzheimer's disease had particular difficulty in understanding familiar phrases and idioms, such as 'loud tie'. The authors' suggestion is that this reflects a difficulty in interpreting abstract meanings.

Taken overall there is consistency in the evidence indicating that comprehension difficulties do occur. The exploration of their exact nature has not proceeded far, although there are suggestions that lexical difficulties may be paramount for the comprehension of written material (Schwartz et al, 1979) and the identification of particular problems in understanding familiar idiomatic phrases.

Other language impairments

Many aspects of language have been poorly explored, but the evidence indicates that most language-related activities show some adverse changes. Writing, repetition of phrases, performance on tests of word fluency, and word association responses have all been shown to be affected by dementia. There is a tendency to perseverate verbal responses (Miller & Hague, 1975; Rosen, 1983; Bayles *et al*, 1985; Pietro & Golfarb, 1985; Ober *et al*, 1986; Grafman *et al*, 1991; Miller & Morris, 1993).

Conclusions

What can be made of the evidence as it stands at present? The work described above, together with other evidence which it has not been possible to include in this paper, points to widespread impairments in language. These include both expressive aspects of language and comprehension of both the written and the spoken word.

There is also evidence that language impairments interact with other types of impairment. An example is the likely role of misperception of the object or picture to be named in explaining some, but not all, errors of naming. As already indicated, it is hardly surprising that such interactions should occur in a condition like Alzheimer-type dementia, which causes such a range of intellectual or cognitive impairments. The difficulty is that these interactions make it more difficult to tease out exactly what is going on within the particular function of interest (in this case, language).

Techniques developed in the study of aphasia have yielded some interesting results, but they beg the question as to whether language deterioration in dementia is really like that in any form of aphasia due to focal lesions. On balance, it appears that dementia does not produce a form of language impairment that is qualitatively the same as that found in any aphasic syndrome associated with focal lesions. However, it is possible that cerebrovascular dementia, with its multiplicity of focal lesions, may produce language impairments that can more accurately be described as aphasic in nature.

As far as the nature of the language impairment in Alzheimer-type dementia is concerned, many strands of evidence point to particular difficulties with the semantic aspects of language and possibly also some difficulties in lexical access. The syntactical and phonological aspects of language appear to remain relatively well preserved. It is always possible to argue that the semantic aspects appear to suffer most, simply because we have more sensitive tests of this aspect of language and that, in any case, the syntactical and phonological aspects may suffer later in the course of the disease. Both are possible, but the fact that it can be relatively easy to detect errors of syntax in some forms of aphasia suggests that the apparent preservation of the syntactical aspects of language in dementia is not merely an artefact of differential test sensitivity. Syntax and phonology may deteriorate markedly in the later stages of dementia, but sophisticated language testing, capable of distinguishing these different aspects, becomes more difficult as the condition progresses.

These comments lead back to the absence of longitudinal studies of language deterioration in dementia. Adverse changes in functioning are progressive in dementia; the process is dynamic and not static. Any full understanding of these changes, whether in language or any other function, must take this progressive aspect into consideration. This demands good longitudinal studies.

Finally, the fact that language impairments occur in dementia means that communication is a problem in the management of people with dementing illnesses. What is also lacking in this area are investigations directed at determining the ways in which some sort of effective communication can best be maintained.

References

APPELL, J., KERTESZ, A. & FISMAN, M. (1982) A study of language functioning in Alzheimer patients. *Brain and Language*, 17, 73–91.
BARKER, M. G. & LAWSON, J. S. (1968) Nominal aphasia in dementia. *British Journal of Psychiatry*, 114, 1351–1356.
BAYLES, K. A. (1982) Language function in senile dementia. *Brain and Language*, 16, 265–280.
—— (1991) Age at onset of Alzheimer's disease: relation to language dysfunction. *Archives of Neurology*, 48, 155–159.
—— & TOMOEDA, C. K. (1983) Confrontation naming in dementia. *Brain and Language*, 19, 98–114.
——, ——, KASZNIAK, A. W., et al (1985) Verbal perseveration of dementia patients. *Brain and Language*, 25, 102–110.
BOWLES, N. L., OBLER, L. K. & ALBERT, M. L. (1987) Naming errors in healthy aging and dementia of the Alzheimer type. *Cortex*, 23, 519–524.
BREITNER, J. C. S. & FOLSTEIN, M. F. (1984) Familial Alzheimer dementia: a prevalent disorder with specific clinical features. *Psychological Medicine*, 14, 63–80.
CODE, C. & LODGE, B. (1987) Language in dementia of recent referral. *Age and Ageing*, 16, 366–372.
CUMMINGS, J. L., BENSON, D. F., HILL, M. A., et al (1985) Aphasia in dementia of the Alzheimer type. *Neurology*, 35, 394–397.
——, HOULIHAN, J. P. & HILL, M. A. (1986) The pattern of reading deterioration in dementia of the Alzheimer's type: observation and implications. *Brain and Language*, 29, 315–323.
DE RENZI, E. & VIGNOLO, L. A. (1962) The token test: a sensitive test to detect receptive disturbances in aphasics. *Brain*, 85, 665–678.

ERNST, B., DALBY, M. A. & DALBY, A. (1970) Aphasic disturbances in presenile dementia. *Acta Neurologica Scandinavica*, **43** (suppl.), 571–576.

FABER-LANGENDOEN, K., MORRIS, J. C., KNESEVICH, J. W., et al (1988) Aphasia in senile dementia of the Alzheimer type. *Annals of Neurology*, **23**, 365–370.

FLICKER, C., FERRIS, S. H., CROOK, T., et al (1987) Implications of memory and language dysfunction in the naming deficit of senile dementia. *Brain and Language*, **31**, 187–200.

GRAFMAN, J., THOMPSON, K., WEINGARTNER, H., et al (1991) Script generation as an indicator of knowledge representation in patients with Alzheimer's disease. *Brain and Language*, **40**, 344–358.

HARTMAN, M. (1991) The use of semantic knowledge in Alzheimer's disease: evidence for impairments of attention. *Neuropsychologia*, **29**, 213–228.

HIER, D. B., HAGENLOCKER, K. & SHINDLER, A. G. (1985) Language disintegration in dementia: effects of etiology and severity. *Brain and Language*, **25**, 117–133.

HUFF, F. J., CORKIN, S. & GROWDON, J. H. (1986) Semantic impairment and anomia in Alzheimer's disease. *Brain and Language*, **28**, 235–249.

HUTCHINSON, J. M. & JENSEN, M. (1980) A pragmatic evaluation of discourse communication in normal and senile elderly in a nursing home. In *Language and Communication in the Elderly* (eds L. K. Obler & M. L. Albert), pp. 59–73. Lexington: Lexington Books.

KEMPLER, D., CURTISS, S. & JACKSON, C. (1987) Syntactic preservation in Alzheimer's disease. *Journal of Speech and Hearing Research*, **30**, 343–350.

——, VAN LANCKER, D. & READ, S. (1988) Proverb and idiom comprehension in Alzheimer's disease. *Alzheimer Disease and Associated Disorders*, **2**, 38–49.

KERTESZ, A., APELL, J. & FISMAN, M. (1986) The dissolution of language in Alzheimer's disease. *Canadian Journal of Neurological Science*, **13**, 415–418.

KIRSCHNER, H. S., WEBB, W. G. & KELLY, M. P. (1984) The naming disorder of dementia. *Neuropsychologia*, **22**, 23–30.

LAWSON, J. S. & BARKER, M. G. (1968) The assessment of nominal dysphasia in dementia. *British Journal of Medical Psychology*, **41**, 411–414.

MARGOLIN, D. I., PATE, D. S., FRIEDRICH, F. J., et al (1990) Dysnomia in dementia and in stroke patients: different underlying cognitive deficits. *Journal of Clinical and Experimental Neuropsychology*, **12**, 597–612.

MARTIN, A. & FEDIO, P. (1983) Word production and comprehension in Alzheimer's disease: the breakdown of semantic knowledge. *Brain and Language*, **19**, 124–141.

MILLER, E. (1989) Language impairment in Alzheimer type dementia. *Clinical Psychology Review*, **9**, 181–195.

—— & HAGUE, F. (1975) Some characteristics of verbal behaviour in presenile dementia. *Psychological Medicine*, **5**, 255–259.

—— & MORRIS, R. (1993) *The Psychology of Dementia*. Chichester: Wiley.

MURDOCH, B. E., CHENERY, H. J., WILLS, V., et al (1987) Language disorder in dementia of the Alzheimer type. *Brain and Language*, **31**, 122–137.

NEBES, R. D., BOLLER, F. & HOLLAND, A. (1986) Use of a semantic context by patients with Alzheimer's disease. *Psychology and Aging*, **1**, 261–269.

NICHOLAS, M., OBLER, L. K., ALBERT, M. L., et al (1985) Empty speech in Alzheimer's disease and fluent aphasia. *Journal of Speech and Hearing Research*, **28**, 405–410.

OBER, B. A., DRONKERS, N. F., KOSS, E., et al (1986) Retrieval from semantic memory in Alzheimer-type dementia. *Journal of Clinical and Experimental Neuropsychology*, **8**, 75–92.

PIETRO, M. J. S. & GOLDFARB, R. (1985) Characteristic patterns of word association responses in institutional elderly with and without senile dementia. *Brain and Language*, **26**, 230–243.

ROCHFORD, G. (1971) A study of naming errors in dysphasic and demented patients. *Neuropsychologia*, **9**, 437–443.

ROSEN, W. A. (1983) Neuropsychological investigation of memory, visuoconstructional, visuoperceptual and language abilities in senile dementia of the Alzheimer type. In *The Dementias* (eds R. Mayeux & W. G. Rosen), pp. 127–141. New York: Raven Press.

SCHWARTZ, M. F., MARIN, O. S. & SFFRAN, E. M. (1979) Dissociations in language function in dementia: a case study. *Brain and Language*, **7**, 277–306.

SELTZER, B. & SHERWIN, I. (1983) A comparison of clinical features in early- and late-onset primary degenerative dementia. *Archives of Neurology*, **40**, 143–146.
SKELTON-ROBINSON, M. & JONES, S. (1984) Nominal dysphasia and severity of senile dementia. *British Journal of Psychiatry*, **145**, 168–171.
STENGEL, E. (1964) Psychopathology of dementia. *Proceedings of the Royal Society of Medicine*, **57**, 911–914.
THOMPSON, I. M. (1987) Language in dementia. *International Journal of Geriatric Psychiatry*, **2**, 145–161.

14 The semantics of autism

PETER HOBSON

This chapter has two aims, as reflected in the ambiguity of its title. The first is to present a thesis about what 'autism' means. The thesis is that autism 'is' the failure to establish patterned interpersonal relatedness with others. The second aim is to illustrate how we can explore this thesis by examining 'word meanings' in the language of autistic people. Over two decades ago, Bosch (1970, p. 61) suggested that with regard to autism, "it is in the language and through the language in particular that the success and failure of the constitution of the common and own worlds are most impressively revealed". I think that Bosch was right: language promises to tell us something about the sources as well as the implications of autistic people's limited experience of self and others as persons-with-mind, and to highlight the resulting handicaps in establishing 'shared meanings' with other people.

In an essay on semantics, Lyons (1987) writes: "Semantics is usually defined by linguists . . . as the study of meaning," and then he qualifies this by stating that most linguists would restrict semantics to the study of meaning in language. He also discusses the difficulties of distinguishing semantics from pragmatics, the focus of which is the use of language in context. One part of such a distinction might be the contrast between linguistic meaning (the meaning of a word, a sentence, etc.) and the *speaker's* meaning in what is being said. As Lyons argues, however, the relation between linguistic expressions and what *they* mean is probably explicable in terms of the relationships among speakers, expressions, and what the speakers mean by the expressions.

We therefore have to be careful about abstracting 'word meanings' from the communicative contexts in which those meanings are learnt. Words are used to express attitudes, they are used in a variety of 'speech acts' to engage with others communicatively (to persuade, to greet, to inform, etc.), and they both embody and effect what we call 'thinking'. It is significant from the developmental perspective that children have to *learn* how words are used meaningfully, and for this they need to have some *pre*-linguistic apprehension of what it means to share and to communicate, and, in due course, what it means to use words 'correctly'. An understanding of *the* meaning of a word involves more than coming to use a particular sound successfully, to get things done – it also entails a grasp of how the meaning that the word has for oneself (whether spoken or comprehended) is also the meaning that the word has for others (Mead, 1934; Kaye, 1982). Once again, a vital route to such understanding is the pre-linguistic infant's ability to discern what someone else is intending to communicate or express by the use of words.

It follows that even before language development 'takes off' around the middle of the second year of life, an infant must *already* sense what it means for people to intend to communicate and to refer to things or events that exist in a shared world. Here we see the need to analyse the roots of language in the forms of interpersonal understanding afforded by infants' non-verbal communication with other people over the first 18 months of life. The need is especially pressing if we are to explain the coincidence between autistic children's profound impairment in affective contact with other people (Kanner, 1943), and their characteristic delays and 'deviance' in language development.

The meaning of 'autism'

If we consider what 'autism' means according to any of the principal diagnostic manuals, we find that it is a syndrome pithily characterised by Lorna Wing (e.g. 1988) as an early-onset disorder in social interaction, social communication, and social imagination and understanding, one that is associated with other features such as repetitive patterns of activity and unusual responses to sensory stimuli. In order to illustrate what this amounts to, and to establish a frame of reference for what follows, I turn to what Kanner meant when he introduced his idea of "autistic disturbances of affective contact" in his seminal paper of 1943. The edited extract below is from his 'Case 9'.

> Charles was brought to the clinic at the age of four and a half years, his mother complaining how "the thing that upsets me most is that I can't reach my baby". As a baby, this child would lie in the crib, just staring. When he was one and a half years old, he began to spend hours spinning toys and the lids of bottles and jars. His mother remarked: "He would pay no attention to me and show no recognition of me if I enter the room. . . . The most impressive thing is his detachment and his inaccessibility. He walks as if he is in a shadow, lives in a world of his own where he cannot be reached. No sense of relationship to persons. He went through a period of quoting another person; never offers anything himself. His entire conversation is a replica of whatever has been said to him. He used to speak of himself in the second person, now he uses the third person at times; he would say, 'He wants' – never 'I want' . . ."

Here we can see what 'autistic' disorder in social interaction and in social communication (both non-verbal and linguistic) amounts to. If one adds that such children are severely restricted in their interpersonal understanding, their creative symbolic play and their imaginative thinking, one has the core of what 'autism' means.

Or do we need to go further than that? I recall having a dispute with an authority on autism, who was arguing that it is a waste of time to dwell on the question 'what is autism?'. One should simply accept that there is a syndrome, a constellation of clinical phenomena, that we choose to name in this way. I disagreed, and I do disagree, in that I believe there is an essence of autism, 'a something' that autism means and that Kanner was trying to capture (Hobson, 1991a). Indeed, not only Kanner but also other clinicians have referred to how the autistic child relates to other people as if they were pieces of furniture. This (oversimplified) characterisation is not simply a detached description – it captures something of what it is like to be in the presence of a severely autistic person, to be treated in some ways *like* a piece of furniture. It is part of one's own experience of being in relation to an autistic person – and it is importantly different to what we normally feel in our interpersonal relations.

This prompts me to reformulate Kanner's thesis about what autism means, or more strongly still, what autism 'is'. The thesis is that autism is a certain kind of failure in interpersonal engagement, most succinctly described as an impairment in the capacity for intersubjective coordination. Normally there are processes that lead to a linkage of subjective experiences across people, processes rooted in basic, animal-level kinds of non-verbal communication and affective responsiveness, but these processes have gone awry in autism. In my view, it is this that gives rise to those impairments characteristic of autism (coincidental mental retardation aside) in interpersonal understanding, in creative symbolic functioning, and in the realm of language (Hobson, 1993). This chapter illustrates this line of thinking by focusing on three separate facets of semantics as applied to the case of autism. These will serve to clarify what Bosch meant in referring to autistic children's difficulty in constituting a world that is held in common with others, but also a world that is one's own.

Suppose for a moment that the thesis about autistic children having a primary incapacity in intersubjective and especially affective interpersonal engagement has some validity. If one adopts the perspective of genetic epistemology, it follows that autistic people should encounter specific difficulty in grasping concepts for which appropriately configured emotional experience is necessary. To oversimplify, if the coordination of emotional experience between autistic children and others is deficient, then these children might be expected to have a specific difficulty in recognising the meaning of those words that have to do with emotion-related concepts. One might predict that even if one took a sample of able autistic children who have acquired quite a lot of language, one would find within that language specific semantic difficulties with words that are 'emotion related' in meaning.

Studies in semantics

'Emotion' words

If autistic children are handicapped in having, expressing and recognising appropriately patterned emotional states in the course of their interpersonal relations, then it is likely that they will also be handicapped in achieving a firm and full understanding of what people mean when they use 'emotion' words such as 'angry' or 'jealous'. Not only will other people feel hesitant and uncertain in using such words about the children's own emotional states if the children express those emotion states in muted or idiosyncratic ways (as they often do: Ricks, 1975; Ricks & Wing, 1975; Langdell, 1981; Macdonald et al, 1989; Dawson et al, 1990; Yirmiya et al, 1991), but so too autistic children will be ill-placed to 'read' the bodily expressed emotions of others (cf. the evidence for emotion recognition deficits in autism, summarised by Hobson, 1991b). Most importantly, they may fail to 'get inside' the subjective states of others in such a way as to identify (and identify *with*) what is being meant when other people use emotion terms about themselves or third parties.

As a first step towards investigating this matter, colleagues and myself pairwise matched 21 autistic and 21 non-autistic retarded adolescents and young adults for chronological age and overall verbal ability (Hobson et al, 1989). We also tested a group of 21 normal young children who were individually matched for verbal mental age.

Subjects were presented with two sets of six photographs of faces. One set showed the faces of a man, and the other set the faces of a woman, with 'standardised' expressions of happiness, unhappiness, fear, anger, surprise and disgust, taken (with permission) from Ekman & Friesen (1975). There were three sets of 'non-emotion' photographs, one depicting vehicles (a bus, a racing car, a milk float, a lorry, an aeroplane, and a dumper-truck), another depicting birds (a seagull, a duck, an owl, a budgerigar, a hen, and a song-thrush), and the third depicting garden tools (a pair of shears, a spade, a rake, a broom, a lawnmower, and an axe). The sets of photographs were presented one at a time, with emotion and non-emotion sets alternating with each other. In each case, the experimenter pointed out that the photographs showed the same person with different feelings, or were all pictures of (for example) vehicles or birds. Subjects were asked to say how the person 'feels' in each picture, or to name the objects depicted, and their responses were recorded verbatim.

In a subsequent session, we presented tape-recorded sounds expressive of each of the emotions, or indicative of each of the non-emotion items that had appeared in the photographs. There were two emotion tapes, one of non-verbal vocalisations (angry snorts and 'grr' sounds, sad sighs and groans, high-pitched tones of fear, etc.) and the other of a neutral passage of prose read in each of the six emotionally expressive tones of voice. The three non-emotion tapes comprised 10-second BBC Sound Library recordings of the vehicles, birds, and gardening tools (e.g. shears clipping, broom sweeping, etc.). The children were asked: "What feeling was that?" and "How did *that* person feel?" in the case of the emotion tapes, and "What bird was that?" and so on when the non-emotion meaningful sounds were presented.

Subjects' responses were transcribed and judged for accuracy (on a scale of 0, inaccurate, to 2, correct and specific) by raters who were 'blind' to the hypothesis underlying the study. The results are illustrated by the scores on naming sounds (Fig. 14.1). The most critical result for the case of autism is the comparison between autistic and non-autistic retarded children, where both for the photographs and for the sounds tasks, there was a significant interaction of group × conditions, with autistic subjects showing specific difficulties in naming emotion items. In keeping with a number of other studies of this kind (e.g. Hobson *et al*, 1988; Ozonoff *et al*, 1990; Prior *et al*, 1990), the group difference was not significant when subjects were compared on emotion items *alone*, but the significant difference emerged when subjects' *profiles* of performance on different forms of task (emotion v. non-emotion) were considered.

'Emotion-related' words

When appraising results from studies with autistic children, it is always important to bear in mind how they have been matched with control subjects. In the studies just described, subjects were matched according to performance on a standard picture-naming task, the British Picture Vocabulary Scale (BPVS; Dunn *et al*, 1982). As we have seen, autistic subjects were not significantly worse than control subjects at naming emotions, when this was considered in isolation with the BPVS as a benchmark. But what kind of 'benchmark' is a language-related task like the BPVS?

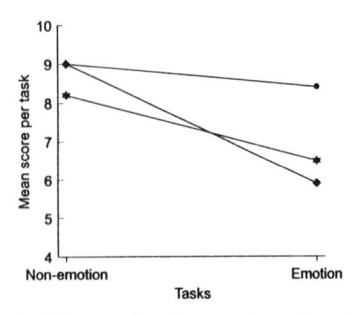

Fig. 14.1. Mean score (range 0–12) on naming of non-emotion and emotion sounds by matched groups of autistic (—◆—), non-autistic retarded (—★—), and normal children (—●—)

The rationale for using such a test to match subjects is that only in this way can one exclude *general* language ability as determining differences between groups on tests requiring language. (In fact, this is not strictly true when there are different profiles in performance across different tasks, as in the present case.) However, in laying the emphasis on linguistic constraints on task performance, such an approach neglects the fact that interpersonal affective coordination may play an influential role in determining language acquisition. In particular, much language is learnt through young children identifying the attitudes and intentions of language users, and identifying *with* those attitudes and intentions in speaking themselves – and *these* abilities and propensities may have much to do with the child's capacities for affect-related psychological engagement with other people (Hobson, 1993). If this is so, then matching on an 'emotion-related' index of cognitive function – in this case, one to do with language – will tend to normalise subjects' performance on at least some 'emotion' tasks.

My colleague Tony Lee and I decided to explore a specific component of this thesis (Hobson & Lee, 1989). Suppose we looked *within* the BPVS itself: when comparing subjects who had similar overall performance on this test, could we find evidence that the most 'emotion-related' items were more difficult for autistic than non-autistic subjects?

On the BPVS, subjects are presented with a series of plates showing drawings arranged in groups of four. Subjects are given instructions such as "Point to . . . dentist", or "Show me . . . surprise," and they respond by indicating the appropriate picture. In order to select emotion-related and emotion-unrelated items for comparison, we asked colleagues who were unaware of the nature of our study to judge whether, in evaluating the meanings of the words with reference to the pictures, their judgements had reference to emotion (on a scale of 0–2). We also asked them to judge the items according to 'abstractness', which (following Paivio *et al*, 1968) we defined as involving concepts that cannot be experienced by the senses. The emotion-related items included word–picture combinations that ranged from 'horror' and 'delighted' to more complex notions like 'greeting' and 'snarling'. Although the majority of these were also included in the list of abstract items, this list also featured non-emotion terms such as 'time', 'pair', and 'adjustable'. Because the items of the test are arranged in order of increasing difficulty, it was possible to compare matched pairs of autistic and non-autistic subjects on emotion-related and emotion-unrelated items that are equally difficult for normal subjects.

As expected, non-autistic retarded subjects achieved similar scores on the selected emotion-related and emotion-unrelated items, but, in contrast, autistic subjects were specifically poorer on the emotion-related items. On the other hand, autistic and non-autistic subjects were equally able to judge non-emotion-related abstract words vis-à-vis equally difficult 'concrete' words. This made it unlikely that the autistic children's difficulties in emotion-related understanding was simply a reflection of the greater abstractness of the words involved. Instead, it seemed that on a linguistic conceptual level, significant group differences were demonstrable specifically in the realm of emotional understanding.

These results do not reveal the source of autistic children's difficulties with emotion-related meanings, and they certainly do not allow one to conclude that some kind of impairment in affective contact is central to the disorder. For example, autistic children are also specifically delayed in appreciating the meanings of other terms referring to mental states, perhaps especially those that have to do with thinking and believing (e.g. Baron-Cohen, 1991). However, the results do contribute to our attempts to map the domain in which autistic children's experience and understanding of mental states seems to be partial.

Personal pronouns

I have claimed that language learning leans heavily on the young child's ability to recognise and identify with the attitudes and intentions in speaking of the people from whom language is learnt (Tomasello, 1992). My final example of language studies in autism exemplifies this close meshing of 'semantic' understanding and interpersonal engagement.

The example concerns the comprehension and use of the personal pronouns 'I' and 'you'. Consider how a child learns to say "I do it" or "I'm hurt" from hearing another person uttering these expressions in appropriate contexts. In order to adopt such utterances themselves when they are doing it or feeling it, children have to understand that such words express the speaker's stance and attitude. When children themselves adopt a similar stance or attitude, they can express similar things in a similar way. Therefore, as de Villiers & de Villiers (1974) point out, 'I' and 'you' are words that can only be understood by 'non-egocentric' people who recognise the context of the relationship between the speaker and the addressee. The reciprocal roles in discourse give meaning to 'I' and 'you'. Such roles have much to do with the fact that self and other are alike insofar as they can have similar attitudes and intentions, but different insofar as any particular attitude or conversational stance may belong to one person at a given time and to another person subsequently. I have already implied that (preverbal) affective coordination may be especially important for children's awareness that they share subjective states with other people. Usage of personal pronouns is a linguistic manifestation of normal two-year-olds' appreciation of the fact that people are also 'selves' with their own subjective orientations.

What, then, of the usage of personal pronouns by children who are delayed in recognising the differentiation and complementarity of self and other? Such children will be likely to associate another person's utterance not with that other person's psychological stance, but rather with the context as experienced by the child. One result is that these children would repeat the utterance as heard when they found themselves in the same situation once again – the 'same situation' being that of the listener in the original context, not in the situation of the speaker who used 'I'. Recall how in Kanner's Case 9 the patient rarely used the personal pronoun 'I', and how he used to speak of himself as 'you' or 'he'. He would also quote (or probably 'echo') other people. In reviewing his series of cases, Kanner wrote:

> "the absence of spontaneous sentence formation and the echolalia type reproduction has, in every one of the eight speaking children, given rise to a peculiar grammatical phenomenon. *Personal pronouns are repeated just as heard*, with no change to suit the altered situation. The child, once told by his mother, 'Now I will give you your milk', expresses the desire for milk in exactly the same words. Consequently, he comes to speak of himself always as 'you', and of the person addressed as 'I'. Not only the words, but even the intonation is retained. . . . There is a set, not-to-be-changed phrase for every specific occasion". (Kanner, 1943, p. 244) (Kanner's emphasis)

Here we see how one possible explanation for the association between echolalia and confusions in the use of personal pronouns is that autistic children fail to identify with the other person who uses the self-expressive 'I'. This would account for the child's failure to adapt speech in appropriate, non-echolalic fashion (also Mahler, 1968; Charney, 1981; Prizant & Wetherby, 1987; see also Bartak & Rutter, 1974; Fay, 1979; for alternative interpretations).

Tony Lee and I, in collaboration with a psycholinguist, Shula Chiat, tested the specific prediction that autistic subjects would differ from matched non-autistic control subjects in either confusing personal pronouns or in avoiding such pronouns by using proper names instead (Lee *et al*, 1993). We studied groups of autistic and non-autistic retarded adolescents who were closely matched for age and verbal ability. To begin with, we ascertained from teachers whether the children had current problems in using personal pronouns. There was not a single non-autistic subject who had such a problem, but according to two independent informants, 17 out of 25 autistic subjects made sporadic errors in this respect. Then, among other tasks, we presented pairs of photographs to subjects, and asked a simple question as the experimenter pointed to each in turn, "Who is this a picture of?", or, in another condition, "Who is wearing the hat/scarf?" Although there were no errors at all in terms of comprehension (e.g. "Point to me/you"), the majority of lower-ability autistic subjects consistently referred to themselves and the experimenter by their proper names, whereas most matched controlled subjects tended to use personal pronouns. In another experiment, we presented each subject with a pile of photographs of peers, inserted among which was a photograph of the subject and another of the experimenter. Instructions were to "Tell me who they are". There was a significant overall group difference, in that the autistic subjects were less likely than non-autistic subjects to call the experimenter 'you', although in this case there was not a statistically significant difference in usage of the first-person pronoun.

Our conclusion from the study (which included other experiments) was that these relatively able autistic children were not so much unable to comprehend and produce pronouns (although we suspect that these do present difficulties for young autistic children), but rather that there were significant group differences in the *propensity* to use such pronouns in certain circumstances, for instance when they were naming themselves and others in photographs. Our tentative interpretation is that autistic subjects' use of names and not pronouns for photographs might have reflected a relatively detached, almost 'third-person' attitude to these pictures of themselves and the experimenter. In contrast, non-autistic subjects seemed to identify with the photographs of themselves, and to see and care about the photographed person as 'me', and to relate to the experimenter as 'you'. These interpretations are far from conclusive, but the approach exemplifies the potential value of studying autistic children's grasp of word meanings as a window on their abnormalities in interpersonal engagement and understanding.

Conclusions

Autism is centrally a problem with intersubjective engagement and coordination between the autistic person and others. The sources of this impairment concern affective relatedness with others; its implications include the capacity to recognise and identify with other people as 'selves' with their own subjective psychological orientations. I have not dealt with a range of additional manifestations in language, especially in the pragmatics of language use, that appear to reflect underlying restrictions in autistic children's experience and understanding of the nature of other persons with whom they can share experiences, and with whom they enter into relations of mutual conflict, agreement, competition, information exchange, and so on (e.g. Bosch, 1970; Hobson, 1993). Already we have learnt much from the study of pragmatic as well as semantic deficits in the language of autistic people (Baltaxe, 1977; Baron-Cohen, 1988; Hobson, 1989; Loveland *et al*, 1989; Wetherby, 1986). Just as language may afford unique insights into autistic people's impoverished experience of the interpersonal world, so autism promises to shed light on the origins and nature of language itself.

References

BALTAXE, C. A. M. (1977) Pragmatic deficits in the language of autistic adolescents. *Journal of Paediatric Psychology*, **2**, 176–180.

BARON-COHEN, S. (1988) Social and pragmatic deficits in autism: cognitive or affective? *Journal of Autism and Developmental Disorders*, **18**, 379-402.

―― (1991) The development of a theory of mind in autism: deviance and delay? In *Psychiatric Clinics of North America*, **14**, 33-51.

BARTAK, L. & RUTTER, M. (1974) The use of personal pronouns by autistic children. *Journal of Autism and Childhood Schizophrenia*, **4**, 217-222.

BOSCH, G. (1970) *Infantile Autism*. New York: Springer-Verlag.

CHARNEY, R. (1981) Pronoun errors in autistic children: support for a social explanation. *British Journal of Disorders of Communication*, **15**, 39-43.

DAWSON, G., HILL, D., SPENCER, A., et al (1990) Affective exchanges between young autistic children and their mothers. *Journal of Abnormal Child Psychology*, **18**, 335-345.

DE VILLIERS, P. A. & DE VILLIERS, J. G. (1974) On this, that, and the other: nonegocentrism in very young children. *Journal of Experimental Child Psychology*, **18**, 438-447.

DUNN, L. M., DUNN, L. M. & WHETTON, C. (1982) *British Picture Vocabulary Scale*. Windsor: NFER-Nelson.

EKMAN, P. & FRIESEN, V. W. (1975) *Unmasking the Face. A Guide to Recognizing Emotions from Facial Clues*. Englewood Cliffs: Prentice-Hall.

FAY, W. H. (1979) Personal pronouns and the autistic child. *Journal of Autism and Developmental Disorders*, **9**, 247-260.

HOBSON, R. P. (1989) Beyond cognition: a theory of autism. In *Autism: Nature, Diagnosis, and Treatment* (ed. G. Dawson), pp. 22-48. New York: Guilford.

―― (1991a) What is autism? *Psychiatric Clinics of North America*, **14**, 1-17.

―― (1991b) Methodological issues for experiments on autistic individuals' perception and understanding of emotion. *Journal of Child Psychology and Psychiatry*, **32**, 1135-1158.

―― (1993) *Autism and the Development of Mind*. Hillsdale: Lawrence Erlbaum.

――, OUSTON, J. & LEE, A. (1988) Emotion recognition in autism: coordinating faces and voices. *Psychological Medicine*, **18**, 911-923.

――, ―― & ―― (1989) Naming emotion in faces and voices: abilities and disabilities in autism and mental retardation. *British Journal of Developmental Psychology*, **7**, 237-250.

―― & LEE, A. (1989) Emotion-related and abstract concepts in autistic people: evidence from the British Picture Vocabulary Scale. *Journal of Autism and Developmental Disorders*, **19**, 601-623.

KANNER, L. (1943) Autistic disturbances of affective contact. *Nervous Child*, **2**, 217-250.

KAYE, K. (1982) *The Mental and Social Life of Babies*. London: Methuen.

LANGDELL, T. (1981) *Face perception: An Approach to the Study of Autism*. Unpublished doctorial thesis, University College, London.

LEE, A., HOBSON, R. P. & CHIAT, S. (1993) I, you, me and autism: an experimental study. *Journal of Autism and Developmental Disorders*, **24**, 155-176.

LOVELAND, K. A., TUNALI, B., KELLEY, M. L., et al (1989) Referential communication and response adequacy in autism and Down's syndrome. *Applied Psycholinguistics*, **10**, 301-313.

LYONS, J. (1987) Semantics. In *New Horizons in Linguistics* (ed. J. Lyons, R. Coates, M. Denchar & G. Gazdar), pp. 152-248. London: Penguin.

MACDONALD, H., RUTTER, M., HOWLIN, P., et al (1989) Recognition and expression of emotional cues by autistic and normal adults. *Journal of Child Psychology and Psychiatry*, **30**, 865-877.

MAHLER, M. S. (1968) *On Human Symbiosis and the Vicissitudes of Individuation*. New York: International Universities Press.

MEAD, G. H. (1934) *Mind, Self and Society*. Chicago: University of Chicago Press.

OZONOFF, S., PENNINGTON, B. F. & ROGERS, S. J. (1990) Are there emotion perception deficits in young autistic children? *Journal of Child Psychology and Psychiatry and Allied Disciplines*, **3**, 343-361.

PAIVIO, A., YUILLE, J. C. & MADIGAN, S. A. (1968) Concreteness, imagery and meaningfulness values for 925 nouns. *Journal of Experimental Psychology* (monograph suppl. 76), 1-25.

PRIOR, M. R., DAHLSTROM, B. & SQUIRES, T.-L. (1990) Autistic children's knowledge of thinking and feeling states in other people. *Journal of Child Psychology and Psychiatry and Allied Disciplines*, **31**, 587-601.

PRIZANT, B. M. & WETHERBY, A. M. (1987) Communicative intent: a framework for understanding social-communicative behavior in autism. *Journal of the American Academy of Child and Adolescent Psychiatry*, **26**, 472–479.

RICKS, D. M. (1975) Vocal communication in pre-verbal normal and autistic children. In *Language, Cognitive Deficits, and Retardation* (ed. N. O'Connor), pp. 75–80. London: Butterworths.

—— & WING, L. (1975) Language, communication and the use of symbols in normal and autistic children. *Journal of Autism and Childhood Schizophrenia*, **5**, 191–221.

TOMASELLO, M. (1992) The social bases of language acquisition. *Social Development*, **1**, 67–87.

WETHERBY, A. M. (1986) Ontogeny of communicative functions in autism. *Journal of Autism and Developmental Disorders*, **16**, 295–316.

WING, L. (1988) The continuum of autism characteristics. In *Diagnosis and Assessment in Autism* (eds E. Schopler & G. B. Mesibov), pp. 91–110. New York: Plenum.

YIRMIYA, N., KASARI, C., SIGMAN, M., *et al* (1989) Facial expressions of affect in autistic, mentally retarded and normal children. *Journal of Child Psychology and Psychiatry*, **30**, 725–735.

15 Growth points in the neurology of speech and language

E. M. R. CRITCHLEY

This chapter discusses those aspects of the neurology of language in which one may expect advances to be made in the near future.

Reception

The receptive aspects of language and speech have been particularly neglected in recent years. Among the *Discources* of Epictetus of Hierapolis is the statement that "Nature has given man one tongue, but two ears, that we may hear twice as much as we speak". This adage is doubly apt in that a child needs the stimulus of heard speech (or alternative forms of communication) to initiate his/her own means of communication. The notion of an innate tendency to speak, as opined by King James I, who thought that a child left to its own devices would speak perfect Hebrew, has no basis in fact. Also, people must constantly monitor their own speech through feedback mechanisms to remove unacceptable intrusions into speech and to ensure the accuracy of what they are saying. Failure to do so may be an early sign of comprehension defects or dementia.

In the absence of reflex encouragement, the babbling of a deaf child dries up (Critchley, 1967a). Because of receptive difficulties the deaf child has problems in acquiring an adequate inner language or vocabulary and experiences difficulties with comprehending concepts, ethics and abstract words (e.g. up, under, above, within) (Critchley, 1967b).

Feedback mechanisms can be examined in a number of ways. I examined the errors made by trainee typists and compared them with those made by experts in the World Speed Championships held in the 1920s at the Old Madison Square Gardens in New York (Critchley, 1968). The transposition and reversal errors made by the sample of trainee typists accounted for 5–7% of all errors made in the World Speed Championships (Book, 1925).

Reversals or transpositions of letters, sounds or words are seen in the initial stages of language acquisition and may persist in dyslexia or as spoonerisms in adult speech. They have been explained as a problem of order or spacing in time (Luchsinger & Arnold, 1965) or of spatial orientation due to delayed maturation of the non-dominant hemisphere (Money, 1962). A better explanation might become available if we accept that:

(a) there is a tendency to make reversals during the learning process for talking, reading and writing
(b) even the most competent will continue to make or overlook errors of transposition in typing or proofreading
(c) such errors are rare when learning to sing or play musical instruments
(d) transposition and reversal errors are closely related to the accuracy of kinaesthetic discrimination.

The differentiation of receptive disorders of speech, especially those due to deafness, from disorders of comprehension is fundamental to the study of learning disorders and also to the recognition of dementia. No study of speech, language or thought disorders in dementia can be said to have a scientific basis unless hearing is specifically examined.

Listening is an active process. Not only does one interpret the words for their meaning but the nuances, emotional inflections, stresses, urgency, sense and manner of the communication. The listener also looks, and may follow the gestures used. For most neonates, children and adults, the face gives an identity, an appearance of intelligence, and a means of communicating emotion. Children with facial agenesis are regarded as unintelligent. Unrecognised facial rigidity in early Parkinsonism results in misread emotions. Schizophrenic people are limited in their ability to interpret facial expression. Lip-reading depends on facial expression as well as lip movement and is difficult if the speaker is hirsute or wears dark glasses (Critchley, 1985).

Central disorders of language

Confirmation of the importance of examining receptive difficulties comes from the fact that at the Psychiatric Unit for the Deaf at Preston patients are occasionally seen with central language disorders masquerading as deafness. Such disorders are complex, fascinating and often multifactorial. There may be a degree of peripheral deafness, or social deprivation, often a change of culture, and other factors such as mental retardation, brain damage, and maturation delay, or psychiatric features can be present. The major syndromes include:

(a) developmental dysphasia
(b) central deafness – failure to perceive the symbolic value of speech sounds, as when listening to an alien language
(c) idiopathic language retardation – often allied to developmental dyslexia and limited gestural ability
(d) word deafness (Worster-Drought & Allen, 1928/29)
(e) word-meaning deafness
(f) auditory phonological agnosia
(g) category-specific access problems (Ellis & Young, 1988)

Pure word deafness can be analysed using dichotic listening techniques. Normally the most active channel involves right-ear preference activating the left-hemisphere language zone. With word deafness this primary system is impaired. The subject can read, write, speak and hear non-speech sounds but is unable to repeat or understand what is said. Vowels are perceived better than consonants. Such difficulties can be partially overcome by slowing the rate of speech to enable the use of alternative pathways as, for example, the right-hemisphere auditory analysis system (Auerbach *et al*, 1982).

Linguistic functions of the right hemisphere

Prosody, the melodic flow and inflection of speech responsive to the phonetic rules and style of a given language or dialect, is a bilateral function with possibly greater input from the right hemisphere. However, it may be surprisingly well preserved in patients who have had split-brain operations, although it is likely that some transference of hemispheric function through plasticity of the nervous system occurred before operation.

It is also accepted that reading involves the non-dominant hemisphere to a greater extent than speech. In deep dyslexia (Coltheart *et al*, 1980), analogous to isolation of the speech area (Geschwind *et al*, 1968), the non-dominant hemisphere is clearly implicated.

Many supralinguistic functions of a cognitive/affective type have been related to the right hemisphere, for example: word-finding, new learning, problem-solving, metaphor interpretation, sentence completion tasks, abstract concepts, story recall, punch-line selection, and verbal humour. Their location and relevance to speech is far from clear.

Lateralisation of speech

The cerebral hemispheres, although apparently similar in structure, are unique among the paired organs of the body in that they differ from each other in their functions, particularly with respect to language and spatial orientation. The cerebral hemispheres appear to adopt simultaneous but distinctive stratagems for processing information (Witelson, 1983). The dominant hemisphere analyses stimuli as discrete items in reference to their temporal arrangement, and the non-dominant hemisphere synthesises stimuli into a unified percept in which the temporal aspects are superseded by spatial relationships.

The concept of laterality for language stems from Broca's observation made in 1865 that most patients with loss of speech have pathological lesions affecting the left hemisphere. Zangwill (1967), in a study of 2133 brain-damaged people, found that 60% of right handers and 55% of left handers with left-hemisphere lesions were aphasic, whereas less than 2% of right handers with right-hemisphere lesions became aphasic. Subsequently, Segalowitz & Bryden (1983), applying Wada's carotid amytal test, found that nearly 20% of left handers showed bilateral language representation. Such people are more liable to suffer aphasia following a stroke, but any aphasia is likely to resolve more readily.

These almost historical observations on handedness and aphasia beg certain questions which have been discussed by Luria (1973):

(a) Is there recovery of injured tissues and reversal of diachisis, allowing return of function?
(b) Is there a shift of function to homologous areas of the other hemisphere?
(c) Does reorganisation occur, permitting entirely different neuronal structures to assume control (as in Goldman's (1972) competition hypothesis)?

A dynamic view of aphasias

The word 'aphasia' is best reserved for acquired disorders of speech, and dysphasia to indicate a developmental impairment of speech (M. Critchley, 1967). Both types of speech disturbance can occur in children. Transitory abnormalities of speech may occur during or immediately following seizures and may occur with a wide variety of seizure type. Acquired aphasia, often with a chronic or progressive course – the Landau–Kleffner syndrome (Landau & Kleffner, 1957) – may occur between the ages of 2 and 13 years. The condition probably does not represent a homogeneous entity; it is relatively rare and hypotheses often relate to a particular observer's limited experience.

Aphasia of Broca's type in childhood usually carries a good prognosis, possibly related to the plasticity of the nervous system. Under 10 years of age most cases resolve within two years. The experience of wartime injuries to the brain (e.g. Mohr *et al*, 1980) suggests that young adults may become aphasic owing to gun-shot wounds over a wide area of the cerebral hemispheres, extending over the recognised inner language zone; most give an aphasia of Broca's type and most tend to recover spontaneously in time.

Exact localisation of speech areas is a myth, although computerised tomography has enabled the accurate identification of lesions affecting interconnecting pathways (i.e. conduction aphasias). Benson's (1979) division of the inner from the outer language zone on the basis of repetition ability, and rostral from caudal lesions on that of fluency, is a useful and practical separation.

It is too easy to regard aphasias as static phenomena, but if examined longitudinally, certain patterns emerge. Global aphasias fare poorly: some may convert to other forms – Broca's, transcortical, conduction, anomic – but few recover completely. Wernicke's aphasia, likewise, has a poor prognosis; but Broca's, conduction, transcortical and anomic aphasias show recovery in 75%, 62%, 50%, and 48% of cases, respectively (Kertesz & McCabe, 1977).

The average age of onset of aphasia deserves consideration. Obler *et al* (1978) found that the median age of presentation was 51 years for Broca's aphasia, 54 for anomic, 56 for global, 57 for conduction, and 63 years of Wernicke's aphasia. Thus, while most aphasias occur around the 50s, Wernicke's aphasia typically occurs 12 years later than Broca's.

Whereas other aphasias represent a limitation of speech, Wernicke's, with its innate fluency, paraphrasia, circumlocutions, neologisms and confabulation, is more accurately defined as a dissolution of speech. Various hypotheses have been proposed to explain the specific nature of Wernicke's aphasia. It is probably not true that with age, strokes occur more posteriorly. Nor, allowing for the fact that aphasic patients lose non-verbal skills, is there a linkage with dementia. But with increasing age there is some loss of plasticity of the brain (i.e. increased differentiation). The most intriguing hypothesis is that Wernicke's aphasia is associated with hormonal or neurotransmitter hypofunction in the elderly.

The neurochemical basis of speech has received scant attention except in animals and birds, many of which are essentially mute save in the mating season. We can detect hormone-related differences in the speech of teenagers and young adults: girls tend to be loquacious, with a high-pitched, rapid speech, and boys' speech tends to be deep, drawled, and monosyllabic.

Anterior language disturbances include Broca's aphasia, frontal alexia (which may overlap with Broca's area), apraxic dysarthria (or cortical articulatory apraxia), and transcortical motor aphasia. The area corresponding to Broca's area on the non-dominant hemisphere has been linked with amusia (Mann, 1898). Trost & Canter (1977) have described an articulatory syndrome of disturbed or inconsistent articulatory performance, impaired speech prosody, an agrammatic, telegraphic style with reduced sentence length, word-finding problems, and impaired (although often mildly so) language comprehension, but many of these symptoms are synonymous with Broca's aphasia.

Various thalamic nuclei, notably the ventrolateral, medial dorsal, anterior and pulvinar, have numerous connections with the speech areas and are linked to aphasic syndromes such as anomia. With the possible exception of Wernicke's aphasia, aphasias are more severe if a cortical lesion is combined with a basal ganglia lesion (Brunner *et al*, 1982), and according to the same authors, automatisms and recurring utterances occur only if there is a combination of cortical and basal ganglia lesions. However, the most common involvement of the thalamus, as evident from stereotactic operations, is an alteration or arrest of the flow of speech. The thalamus shows an asymmetry of function similar to that of the language zones, and appears to be involved in the filtering and focusing of organised verbal codes and in the automatic execution of learned motor plans. Some selective modification also occurs at thalamic level, with the integration of emotional, conceptual, auditory, visual, servokinetic and memory information.

Inner language

We can anticipate a forthcoming book by Frank Benson on Thinking (Oxford University Press). Many strides have been made into memory and the accessibility of memory stores, but the question of inner language, its content and vehicular basis still defies definition. The vehicular basis has been described in terms of a word schema (Brain, 1961), *Vorgestalt* (Conrad, 1954), or preverbitum (M. Critchley, 1967), but these evoke comparisons with the concrete visualisation of the eidetic person and the sketchy silhouettes used by most adults. Whether such an analogy is true we do not know.

The German neurologist Bay (1962) drew attention to the fact that aphasias differ from country to country, reflecting the grammatical and syntactical basis of each language. Indeed, the personality of a fluent polyglot may alter in adaptation to the prosody of a language, the use of gesture and accentuation, of polite if redundant phraseology, and profanities. Bay's other major contribution has been to emphasise that aphasic people perform poorly on non-verbal tasks: that they are "lame in thought" (Bay, 1962).

The frontal lobes and speech

The frontal lobes bring together parts of the evolutionarily older cortex linked to the limbic system with a considerable growth of neocortex, not present in most mammals, recognisable in primates, but accounting for 24% of the neocortex of man. These areas show late maturation, suggestive of much functional sophistication. For many years the frontal cortex was regarded as a silent area of the brain, but its importance gradually became apparent as the result of testing various delayed responses. It is the centre for the construction and monitoring of conscious activity representing many metafunctions: awareness of being aware, self-regulation, motoricity, intentionality, creativity, goal-directed tasks, complex sequencing, and planning. Furthermore, there is evidence of asymmetric activity of the frontal lobes, with dominant hemispheric bias.

Luria (1980) outlined the functions of the frontal lobes as:

(a) regulation of the active state of the subject
(b) control of the essential elements of intentions
(c) programming and execution of complex sequences of actions.

He felt that such self-regulation was dependent on verbal processes; thus patients with frontal lobe lesions can repeat but not follow verbal messages.

Kesner (1985) has added the involvement of short-term memory in information processing on the basis of expectancy. However, an equally important function appears to be the control (or inhibition, or gating) of interference during conscious acts.

Each area of the frontal cortex is closely linked to the appropriate thalamic nuclei, including those already known to be involved in speech processing. Thus the precentral cortex and supplementary motor region project to the ventrolateral nuclei, the prefrontal and orbitofrontal to the medial dorsal, and the integrative and cingulate cortex to the anterior nuclei.

Brown (1985) has defined various syndromes due to lesions of the frontal lobes. Impairment of the left dorsolateral region may show as difficulty in processing verbal messages, facilitating verbal instructions and behavioural tasks. Sentences are shortened and perseveration common. A similar lesion in the left orbitofrontal region will affect ongoing activity, with failure to monitor interference and consequent digression or confabulation. Right frontal lesions (i.e. non-dominant) may influence the final implementation of verbal tasks, with dyspraxia, misarticulation, displacement, or misinterpretation.

Another approach to frontal lobe function is developmental. Vygotsky (1962) observed children performing complex tasks and noted the social interaction between children and adults. The adult gives the child the necessary instructions. The child in performing the task gives him/herself the commands aloud and later plans actions through inner speech. Such behaviour, it is claimed, does not play a regulatory role in mentally retarded children.

Szuman (1985) claims that programmed actions are formulated and perfected only after a child is able to put intentions into words and thus develop a means by which to follow through the intention. This ability to use the regulatory role of verbal instruction is effected in most children between the ages of five and six years, when the frontal lobes attain the first stage of their myelination (Kaczmarek, 1987).

TABLE 15.1
Percentage increases in blood flow in different brain areas on initiating propositional and non-propositional speech

Area	Propositional	Non-propositional
Right supplementary motor region	11%	12%
Right (Broca's) analogue	9%	0%
Right motor cortex	20–30%	20–30%
Left supplementary motor region	26%	19%
Broca's area	21%	0%
Left motor cortex	20–30%	20–30%

The developmental approach is epitomised by an experiment conducted by Luria & Yudovich in 1956. Five-year-old monozygotic twins who did not communicate with anyone except between themselves by means of an idioglossia were separated and placed in different classes. Speech then developed rapidly, so that after ten months not only did they acquire normal speech but they were able to perform complex intellectual tasks. One of the twins (the subordinate one) was given special language training. This brother became the organiser of their planned games. While the trained brother was able to repeat stories, the untrained brother could only answer questions. When classifying objects, the untrained brother grouped a picture of a carrot with a picture of a tram because they were both reddish. The trained brother, on the other hand, formed groups representing fruits, animals, vehicles, and so on.

Initiation of speech

Positron emission tomography offers the expectation of a more thorough and logical examination of the initiation of speech (Ojemann, 1992). It is possible to compare the increase in percentage blood flow during propositional and non-propositional speech (Table 15.1). In effect with propositional speech there is continual activity from the left supplementary motor region initiating speech and gating other signals; activity spreads to Broca's area and thence bilaterally to both motor cortices. With non-propositional speech there is a brief burst from the left supplementary motor region and of activity in Broca's area, after which the motor cortices appear to act independently, probably through thalamic programmes.

References

AUEREBACH, S. H., ALLARD, T., NAESER, M., et al (1982) Pure word deafness: an analysis of a case with bilateral lesions and a defect at the prephonemic level. *Brain*, **105**, 271–300.
BAY, E. (1962) Aphasia and non-verbal disorders of language. *Brain*, **85**, 412–426.
BENSON, D. F. (1979) *Aphasia, Alexia and Agraphia*. Edinburgh: Churchill Livingstone.

BOOK, W. F. (1925) *Learning to Typewrite, with a Discussion of the Psychology and Pedagogy of Skill.* New York: Gregg.
BRAIN, W. R. (1961) *Speech Disorders: Aphasia, Apraxia and Agnosia.* London: Butterworth.
BROWN, J. W. (1985) Frontal lobe syndromes. In *Handbook of Clinical Neurology* (eds G. W. Bruyn & P. J. Vinken), pp. 23–41. Amsterdam, Elsevier.
BRUNNER, R. J., KORNHUBER, H. H., SEEMULLER, E., et al (1982) Basal ganglia participation in language pathology. *Brain and Language*, **16**, 281–299.
COLTHEART, M., PATTERSON, K. & MARSHALL, J. C. (1980) *Deep Dyslexia.* London: Routledge & Kegan Paul.
CONRAD, K. (1954) New problems in aphasia. *Brain*, **77**, 491–509.
CRITCHLEY, E. M. R. (1967a) Hearing children of deaf parents. *Journal of Laryngology and Otology*, **81**, 51–61.
—— (1967b) The social development of deaf children. *Journal of Laryngology and Otology*, **81**, 291–307.
—— (1968) Reversals in language: the importance of kinaesthetic feedback mechanisms. *Journal of Learning Disabilities*, **1**, 32–35.
—— (1985) The human face. *British Medical Journal*, **291**, 1222–1223.
CRITCHLEY, M. (1967) Aphasiological nomenclature and definitions. *Cortex*, **111**, 3–25.
ELLIS, A. W. & YOUNG, A. W. (1988) *Human Cognitive Neuropsychology.* Hove: Lawrence Erlbaum.
GESCHWIND, N., QUADFASEL, F. A. & SEGARRA, J. M. (1968) Isolation of the speech area. *Neuropsychologia*, **6**, 327–340.
GOLDMAN, P. S. (1972) Developmental determinants of cortical plasticity. *Acta Neurobiologiae Experimentalis*, **32**, 495–511.
KACZMAREK, B. L. J. (1987) Regulatory function of the frontal lobes: a neurolinguistic perspective. In *The Frontal Lobes Revisited* (eds E. Perecman), pp. 225–240. London: Lawrence Erlbaum.
KERTESZ, A. & MCCABE, P. (1977) Recovery patterns and prognosis in aphasia. *Brain*, **100**, 1–18.
KESNER, R. P. (1985) Correspondence between humans and animals in coding of temporal attributes. *Annals of the New York Academy of Sciences*, **444**, 122–136.
LANDAU, W. M. & KLEFFNER, F. R. (1959) Syndrome of acquired aphasia with convulsive disorder in children. *Neurology*, **7**, 523–530.
LUCHSINGER, R. & ARNOLD, G. E. (1965) *Voice, Speech, Language.* London: Constable.
LURIA, A. R. (1973) *The Working Brain.* New York: Basic Books.
—— (1980) *Higher Cortical Functions in Man* (2nd edn, revised) (trans. B. Haigh). New York: Basic Books.
—— & YUDOVICH, F. J. (1956) *Speech and Development of Psychological Processes in a Child.* Moscow: Moscow University Press.
MANN, L. (1898) Casuistische Beitrrage zur Hirnchirurgie und Hirnlocalization. *Monatschrift für Psychologie und Neurologie*, **4**, 369–378.
MOHR, J. P., WEISS, G. H., CAVENESS, W. F., et al (1980) Language and motor disorders after penetrating head injury in Vietnam. *Neurology*, **30**, 1273–1279.
MONEY, J. (1962) *Reading Disability – Progress and Research Needs in Dyslexia.* Baltimore: Johns Hopkins Press.
OBLER, L. K., ALBERT, M. L., GOODGLASS, H., et al (1978) Aphasia types and aging. *Brain and Language*, **6**, 318–322.
OJEMANN, G. (1922) Localisation of language in frontal cortex. In *Advances in Neurology* (eds P. Chauvel, A. V. Delgado-Escueta, et al), pp. 361–368. New York: Raven Press.
SEGALOWITZ, S. J. & BRYDEN, M. P. (1983) Individual difference in hemispheric representation of language. In *Language Functions and Brain Organisation* (ed. S. J. Segalowitz), pp. 341–367. London: Academic Press.
SZUMAN, S. (1985) *Selected Works.* Warsaw: Wydawnictwa Szkolne Pedagogiczne.
TROST, J. E. & CANTER, G. L. (1977) Apraxia of speech in patients with Broca's aphasia. *Brain and Language*, **1**, 63–79.
VYGOTSKY, L. S. (1962) *Thought and Language.* Cambridge, MA: MIT Press.

WITELSON, S. F. (1983) Bumps in the brain: right–left asymmetry as a key to functional lateralisation. In *Language Function and Brain Organisation* (ed. S. J. Segalowitz), pp. 117–144. London: Academic Press.

WORSTER-DROUGHT, C. & ALLEN, I. M. (1928/29) Congenital auditory imperception. *Journal of Neurology and Psychopathology*, **60**, 193–289.

ZANGWILL, O. L. (1967) Speech and the minor hemisphere. *Acta Neurologica Belgica*, **67**, 1013–1017.

Further reading

CRITCHLEY, E. M. R. (1987) *Language and Speech Disorders: a Neurophysiological Approach*. London: CNS Press.

PERECMAN, E. (ed.) (1987) *The Frontal Lobes Revisited*. London: Lawrence Erlbaum.

Index

Compiled by STANLEY THORLEY

abstraction and concretism: Holm-Hadulla, H. et al 143
abstractness: autism 179–180
adhesiveness of experience 8, 148–150 & Fig. 12.1, 156–157
adolescent language 140
African languages: syntax influenced by pragmatism 47
alalia: Falret, J. 18–20
Alzheimer's disease,
  introduction 8–9, 14
  language disorder in dementia 163–164, 169–170
  performance on Hodges generations of definitions 77–78 & Fig. 6.2
American/British English: divergences 47
analyses, statistical *see* cluster, covariance, discourse, discriminant function *and* variance
analyses of variance
  language impairments and executive dysfunction 62 & Tab. 5.3
  semantic processing and categorisation 130
analysis of covariance: syntactic processing 102–104
analysis of language
  linguistic performance: Morice, R. 6, 58–62 & Figs 1–2 & Tabs 1–2
  schizophrenic speech: Chaika, E. 5, 47–56
  terminology and techniques: Newby, D. 5, 31–43
  see also computer assistance, cohesion, discourse, psychoanalysis *and* text
anaphora 50
Andreasen, N. J. C.
  formal thought disorder 70
  subtypes of thought disorder 81
  tangentionality 85
anthropological phenomenology: Heidelberg school 138
antonymy: opposite speech 54, 85
aphasia
  19th century views 15–18
  cultural differences 190

differences from schizophrenic speech 71–72
dynamic view 188–190
early interpretations 57–58
global 165, 190
incidence in left and right-handers 188
inner language 190
language impairment in dementia 165–167, 170
similarities to schizophrenic speech 82
transcortical sensory 165–166
aphemia: conceptual history 18–19
articulation: 19th century 17–18
assessments: Comprehensive Assessment of Symptoms and History (CASH) 72, 75–76, 78, 128
associationism: conceptual history 4, 16–17, 23, 25, 27
associations, semantic or phonological 49
asyndesis; Cameron, N. 72
attention: reverse digit span test 102, 104–105 & Tab. 8.4
Austin, J. L.
  negative concepts 155
  'speech acts' 42
autism: semantics 9, 174–184
Ayer, A. J.: Descartes' *cogito* 148

background: speech and language disorders 3–43 Part I
  conceptual history: Berrios, G. 15–30
  introduction: Sims, A. 3–14
  terminology and techniques: D. Newby 31–43
basic definitions 31–32
batteries
  Boston Diagnostic Aphasic Battery 119
  Hodges semantic battery 6, 76–79
  see also scales *and* tests
Begriffsvermögen 83 & Fig. 7.1, 90 & Fig. 7.3, 92–94 & Fig. 7.4
Bentall, R. P.: future research 108
Berrios, G., conceptual history 4, 15–30
Blankenburg, W.: preverbal thinking and predicative language 139–140, 143–144

195

Bleuler, E.
  'loosening of associations' 72, 74
  meanings of neologisms 86
  schizophrenia 23–24
  thought disorder 57–58, 81
Bobon, J.: illustrative case: glossolalia 91
Bosch, G.: word meanings in autism 174, 176
Boston Diagnostic Aphasic Battery 119
brain
  imaging studies 65–66
  localisation: conceptual history 16, 20, 25
  see also Alzheimer's disease, cerebral hemispheres and lesions, frontal lobe syndromes, split-brain operations and thalamic nuclei
British Picture Vocabulary Scale (BPVS) 178–179
British/American English: divergences 47
Broca's aphasia
  language impairment and executive dysfunction 57, 62, 65
  lesions mostly of left hemisphere 188
  prognosis 188–189
  syntactic aspects 169
Brown, J. W.: syndromes due to frontal lobe lesions 191

Cambridge Encyclopaedia of Language (Crystal, 1987) 39
Cameron, N.: overinclusive thinking 115–116
cases, illustrative
  adhesiveness of experience 148–149 & Fig. 12.1
  autism: Kanner, L. 175–176, 181
  development of schizophasic talk in an interview 141–142
  glossolalia: Lecours, A. R. 91–92
  glossomanic utterances 87–89
  morbid speech phenomena: Winslow, F. 18
  thought insertion 11–12, 148–149, 154
catatonic signs: Modified Rogers Scale 128
categorisation: semantic processing 7, 126–137
  conclusions 135
  empirical study 128–131
  theoretical issues and computer simulation model 131–135
central disorders of language 186–187
'central thinking function' 72
cerebral blood flow
  propositional and non-proposional speech 192 & Tab. 15.1
  reduced in chronic schizophrenia 66
cerebral hemispheres
  deficient reciprocal action 19
  dominant 9, 188
  linguistic functions of the right 187
  non-dominant 9, 187–188
cerebral lesions
  posterior cerebral 123
  stroke, left inferior parietal 82
cerebrovascular dementia 9, 170
Chaika, E.
  analysis of schizophrenic speech 47–56
  glossomania: syntactically valid utterances 87
  introduction 5, 12
  random triggering of words and inappropiate perseveration 107
Chen, E. et al: semantic processing and categorisation 7, 13, 126–137
children
  concept construction 33
  deafness 185
  first stage of myelination in frontal lobes (5–6 years) 191
  five-year-old monozygotic twins: language training experiment 192
  language development (two-year-olds) 175
  usage of personal pronouns 180
Chomsky, A. N.
  'deep' structure of sentences 37
  grammar: definition 36
  'linguistic competence' and 'linguistic performance' 61
  sentence: definition 32
classification system of speech acts: Habermas, J. 139
cloze procedure: analysis of information content and redundancy 115
cluster analysis: Tamlyn, D. et al's study 75 & Fig. 6.1
cognitive flexibility: executive impairment 63–64 & Tabs 5.4–5.5, 67
cognitive psychology 127
cohesion analysis 39–40
cohesive ties
  Chaika, E. 50–51
  McKenna, P. 116
  Thomas, P. & Leudar, I. 107
communication
  introduction 3, 7
  syntactic processing in first-onset schizophrenia: Thomas, P. & Leudar, I. 96–112
comprehension: language disorder in dementia 169–170

Comprehensive Assessment of Symptoms and History (CASH)
  categorisation in schizophrenia 128
  language disorder and semantic memory 72, 75–76, 78
computer-assisted analyses
  linguistic impairments: Morice, R. 58–59 & Fig. 5.1
  suite of programs: *PSYCHLAN* 58
  techniques: Newby, D. 38 & Fig. 3.4
computerised tomography 189
concepts
  availability of definitions 152
  construction: opposition impaired in deaf children 33
  negatives 155
conceptual history: Berrios, G. 15–30
  conclusions 26–27
  early descriptions of thought disorder 18–20
  Jackson's views on thought and language 20–21
  Masselon and 'thought disorder' 23
  19th century psychiatric views on thinking and language 16–17
  relationship between thought and language 17–18
  return of the holistic approach 25–26
  Séglas and his book 21–23
  views on thought disorder after Masselon 23–25
conclusions
  analysis of schizophrenic speech 55
  conceptual history 26–27
  German concepts of schizophrenic language disorder 144–145
  introduction 13–14
  language disorder in dementia 170–171
  language disorder and semantic memory 79
  language impairments and executive dysfunction 66–67
  schizophasia 94
  schizophrenic thought and speech 122–123
  semantic processing and categorisation 135
  thought insertion, insight and Descartes' *cogito* 157–158
concretism
  interpretations of delusions 140–141
  Goldstein, K. & Scheerer, M. *Abstract and Concrete Behaviour* 143
consonants: perception better with vowels 187
'conversational implicature': Grice, H. P. 41

conversational speech
  language disorder in dementia 168–169
  necessary functions 71
correlations
  linguistic variables 59–64 & Tabs 5.1–5.4
  thought disorder with percentage errors: study 2 (Mortimer, A. *et al*) 77
  written language study 103–105
Critchley, E. M. R.: neurology of speech and language 9, 185–194
Crow, T. J.: type I and type II schizophrenia 58
Crystal, D.
  definitions 32
  levels 34–36 & Fig. 3.2
Cutting, J.: neuropsychology 118–119
Cutting, J. & Murphy, D.: types of thought disorder 72–73

day dreams 33
deafness
  concept construction in children 33
  differentiation of receptive disorders 9, 186
  major syndromes: Psychiatric Unit for the Deaf at Preston 186–187
definitions
  basic 31–32
  formal thought disorder 70
  grammar 36
  sentences 36–37
delusions
  concretism centering on pre-predicative utterances 7, 140–141
  introduction 7, 10, 14
  psychopathology: intentionality 140, 155
dementia
  aphasia and language impairment 165–166
  aspects of language disorder 9–10, 163–173
  cerebrovascular 9, 170
  recognition 186
dementia praecox
  conceptual history 23–24, 27
  introduction 4
  see also schizophrenia
Descartes' *cogito*, thought insertion and insight 147–159
  adhesiveness 156–157
  "cogito ergo sum" 7–8, 147
  thought insertion 148–150 & Fig. 12.1
diagnoses: DSM-II & DSM-III 50
Discourses of Epictetus of Hierapolis: listening 185

discourse analysis 39–40
discourse level: Rochester, S. & Martin J. R. 115–116
discriminant function analysis: linguistic measures 38
discussion: syntactic processing in first-onset schizophrenia 105–108
'disorganisation syndrome': Liddle, P. F. 73
dominance (cerebral hemispheres) 9, 187–188
DSM–II & DSM–III diagnoses 50
DSM–III
  Australian studies 59
  psychotic/non-psychotic distinction 151
dysarthria 70–71
dysconversation 72–73
dyslalia: conceptual history 22
dyslogia
  Cutting, J. & Murphy, D. 72–73
  Séglas J. 21–22
dysphasia
  comparison with thought disorder 121–122 & Tab. 9.3
  conceptual history 22
  developmental impairment 188
  introduction 3

ego boundaries: introduction 7, 9–13
elderly
  brain-damaged polyglots: glossolalia 94
  controls: Hodges generations of definitions 77 & Fig. 6.2
emotions in autism
  'emotion' words 177–178 & Fig. 14.1
  'emotion-related' words 178–180
  introduction 9
empirical studies
  categorisation 128–131 & Figs 10.1–10.2
  schizophrenic speech 50–52
English
  American/British divergences 47
  syntax influenced by pragmatism 47
epilepsy, temporal lobe: 'forced thoughts' 150–151, 153–154 & Tab. 12.1
errors
  a chronic schizophrenic patient with posterior cerebral lesion-type errors: Shallice, T. *et al* 123
  differences between schizophrenia and mania 51
  numbers in schizophrenic/control groups 59–61 & Fig. 5.2
evaluation: High Royds Evaluation of Negativity 128

evolutionary theory: conceptual history 15
executive dysfunction
  introduction: Sims, A. 6, 12
  language impairments in schizophrenia: Morice, R. 57–69
  slips of the tongue: Chaika, E. 52, 55
exophora 50

Faber, R. & Reichstein, M. B.: language test scores 119–120 & Tab. 9.3
Faber, R. *et al*: thought disorder and dysphasia 121–122 & Tab. 9.3
face photographs: recognition by autistics 177–178
faculty psychology: conceptual history 4, 16–17
Falret, J.: alalia 19–20
feedback mechanisms 185
first rank symptoms: Schneider, K. 10–11, 14
first-onset schizophrenia: syntactic processing and communication disorder 96–112
form (structure): linguistics 35–37 & Figs 3.2–3.3
formal thought disorder
  psychology 114–118, 122–123
  speech 32
forward planning: executive impairment 63–64 & Tabs 5.4–5.5, 67
  Tower of London: Shallice, T. 63
French: syntax influenced by pragmatism 47
Frith, C. D.
  failure of 'meta-representation' 73–74
  'second order representation' (semantic memory) 74
frontal lobes
  first stage of myelination in children (ages 5–6 years) 191
  speech 190–192
  syndromes due to lesions 191
'frontal/executive' rehabilitation programme 66–67
Fulford, W.: thought insertion, insight and Descarte's *cogito* 7–8, 11, 147–159
Furth, H. G.: concept construction in deaf children 33

Garrett, M.: model of sentence production 106–107
Gazzaniga, M.: modular nature of the mind 52
George, L. & Neufeld, R. J. W.: 'loosening of associations' 74

German concepts of schizophrenic language disorder: Mundt, C. 7, 138–146
  conclusions 144–145
  normal speech and language functions 139–141
  phenomenological approaches 141–144
Gestalt paradigms
  schizophrenic thinking 25–26
  worn-out language – novel modes of expression 140
global aphasia 165
  prognosis 189
glossolalia 6, 82, 90–94 & Fig. 7.4
glossomania 6, 82, 84–90 & Fig. 7.3, 93–94
  chains: Chaika, E. 51, 53–54
  composed morphemic deviations 85
  derived morphemic deviations 84–85
  schizographia 89
  utterances 86–90
grammars 35–37 & Figs 3.2–3.3
  transformational or generative 37–39 & Fig. 3.4
Grice, H. P.: conversational 'implicature' and maxims 41
Griesinger W.
  deficient reciprocal act of the two halves of the brain 19
  delusions and obsessions 19
growth points: neurology of speech and language 185–194
Guislain, J.: *d'incohérence des idées* 19

Habermas, J.: classification system of speech acts 139
hallucinations: introduction 10–11, 14
hebephrenics in psychotherapy: 'pernicious fusion' with mother (Lang, H.) 142
Heidelberg school: psychiatric research 138, 143–144
hemispheres *see* cerebral hemispheres
High Royds Evaluation of Negativity: negative symptoms 128
historicism: conceptual history 15–16
history, conceptual: Berrios, G. 4, 15–30
Hobson, P.: semantics of autism 9, 174–184
Hodges, J. R.: semantic impairment in Alzheimer's disease 77 & Fig. 6.2
Hodges semantic battery 6, 76–79
holistic approach: thought disorder (20th century) 25–26
Holm-Hadulla, H. *et al*: abstraction and concretism 143

Hume, D.: personal identity 156–157
Hunt test 6–7, 108–110 App. 1
  complexity variables 100–101, 108–109
  error variables 101, 109–110
  modifications: Hoffman, R. *et al* 100
  syntactic processing in first-onset schizophrenia 97–8, 100–107
  voice (passive/active) 110
hyperphasia 90
hypogeometric distribution 101, 110–111 App. 2
hysteria: Jung, C. G. (conceptual history) 24

ICD-9 & ICD-10: psychotic/non-psychotic distinction 151
"Ice Cream Story": Chaika, E. 50–51, 54
inner language 190
insight
  aphasia and schizophrenia 6, 71–72
  philosophy of mind 8, 152–155 & Tab. 1
  thought insertion 150–152
  thought insertion and Descartes' *cogito* 147–159
intentionality in schizophrenia 140, 143
  investigation of intention 49–50
interfaces
  linguistics/psychiatry 31
  use/structure of language 36 Fig. 3.2, 40–41
interpretations, early: language impairments 57–58
introduction: descriptive pychopathology 3–14
  background 4–5
  conclusions 13–14
  other psychiatric disorders 8–9
  permeability of self 9–13
  schizophrenic disturbance 5–8
Inuits: diversity of words for 'snow' 34

Jackson, H.: thought and language 17, 20–21
  propositions 20
Janzarik, W.: structural-dynamic anthropology 142–143
Jaspers, K.
  comprehending psychology 138
  conceptual history: speech disorders in the psychoses 25
  introduction: self awareness 10
Juliard, P.: interdependence of language and thought 17–18
Jung, C. G.: dementia praecox and hysteria 24–25

Index

Kanner, L.: autism 175–176, 181
Kant, I.: personal identity 156–157
Kasanin, J. & Lewis, N. C. D.: meanings of schizophrenic speech (conceptual history) 25–26
Kesner, R. P.: short-term memory 191
King James I: innate tendency to speak 185
Kleist, K.
    functional disturbances of the temporal speech area 25
    schizophrenic symptoms and cerebral pathology 58
knowledge: equates with semantic memory 74
Kolmogorov-Smirnov goodness-of-fit test 102
Kraepelin, E.
    anatomical perspective 57–58
    'drivelling dementia' 123
    schizophasia 82
Kruskall-Wallis one-way analysis of variance 102, 104 Tab. 8.3 & n.

Lacan, J.: feelings need representation in symbols 142
Landau-Kleffner syndrome 188
language
    central disorders 186–187
    functions and their disturbance 139–141
    inner language 190
language disorder in dementia: Miller, E. 163–173
    aphasia and language impairment 165–166
    comprehension 169–170
    conclusions 170–171
    conversational speech 168–169
    methodological problems 163–164
    naming 166–168
    nature of language impairment 164–165
    other language impairments 170
language disorder and semantic memory: Mortimer, A. et al 70–80
    conclusions 79
    linguistic problems and thought disorder 70–72
    thought disorder as a cognitive dysfunction 72–79
language disorders
    background 1–3 Part I
    psychiatric disorders (non-schizophrenic) 161–194 Part III
    schizophrenic disturbances 45–159 Part II

language impairments
    age of onset 164–165
    related activities 170
language impairments and executive dysfunction: Morice, R. 57–69
    early interpretations 57–58
    executive impairment 62–66 & Tabs 5.4–5.5
    linguistic performance 58–62 & Figs 5.1–5.2 & Tabs 5.1–5.4
langue, pure: opposed to *parole* 48
lateralisation of speech 187–188
Lausanne examples: glossomanic utterances 87–88
Lecours, A.: schizophasia 6, 81–95
Lecours, A. R. & Vanier-Clement, M.: paraphasias 121
levels of linguistic analysis 35–37 & Figs 3.2–3.3
Levy-Valensi, J. *et al*: glossomanic utterances 87–89
Lewis, A.: psychopathology of insight 151–153, 157
lexemes: basic semantic units 39
Liddle, P. F. 'disorganisation syndrome' 73
linguistics
    analysis of schizophrenic speech 47–48, 55 & n.
    analytical levels 35–37 & Figs 3.2–3.3
    discrimination between schizophrenic, manic and control subjects 59
    functions of the right hemisphere 187
    philosophical definitions 152
    problems and thought disorder 70–72
    terminology and techniques 31–43
Lishman, A. W.: 'forced thoughts' 150–151
listening 186
Locke, J.: personal identity 157
logophonic lexicons: input and output 83 & Fig. 7.1
'loosening of associations'
    Bleuler, E. 72, 74
    George, L. & Neufeld, R. J. W. 74
Lordat, J.: 'cascade-type' account of language psychology 17
Luria, A. R.
    functions of the frontal lobes 191
    handedness and aphasia 188

McGrath, J.: model of thought disorder 73
Mackay, D.: schizophrenic errors 52–53

McKenna, P.: schizophrenic thought and speech 7, 13, 113-125
Maher, B.
  distinction between thought and speech models 32-33
  schizophrenic utterances 49 & n.
  semantic priming paradigm 144
Malinowski, B.: phatic communication 34
mania
  diagnosis 50
  error variables: hypergeometric probability 101
  Hunt test 97-98
  linguistic profiles between schizophrenia and normality 59
  similar to schizophrenia with more complex clause structures 97
  types of errors 50
Mann-Whitney test 102, 104
Masselon, P.: *Psychologie des Déments Précoces* 16, 23-24
meaning
  'autism' 175-177
  'meaning' 38-39
medical models 152-154
memory
  episodic 74
  impairment studies in schizophrenia: Tamlyn, D. *et al* 72-79
  long-term 74
  semantic 6-7, 70-80
  short-term 65, 101, 191
  working 7, 12, 65, 101-102, 104-106 & Tab. 8.4
'meta-representation': Frith, C. D. 73-74
metaphors
  emphasis on meanings 47-48
  loss of authenticity 140
methodological problems: language disorder in dementia 163-164
Miller, E.: language disorder in dementia 8-9, 163-173
mimicry, disturbances: Séglas, J. 22
mirror derivations: glossomanic utterances 89 & Fig. 7.2
models
  19th century 16-17
  distinction between thought and speech: Maher, B. 32-33
  evolutionary 25
  glossolalic schizophasia 92-93 & Fig. 7.4
  glossomanic schizophrenia 90 & Fig. 7.3
  Hoffman/Garrett 107
  information processing 19
  medical 152-154
  neural network simulation 128, 133-135 & Figs 10.4-10.5
  parallel-distributed: mental representations 132
  property comparison: categories 132
  sentence production: Garrett, M. 106-107
  speech 83-84 & Fig. 7.1
  thinking 16-17
  thought disorder: McGrath, J. 73
  two-stage feature comparison: semantic processing 132
  what model?: Chaika, E. 45-46
Modified Rogers Scale: catatonic signs 128
Montgomery-Asberg scale: mood state 128
mood state: Montgomery-Asberg scale 128
Morice, R.: language impairments and executive dysfunction 6, 57-69
morphemes
  composed deviations 85
  derived deviations 84-85
  schizophrenic 54
  smallest units of grammar 36
morphology 36 & Fig. 3.2
  free: glossomanic utterances 88-89
Mortimer, A. *et al*: language disorder and semantic memory 6, 12, 70-80
Müller, M.: thought and language inseparable 18
multiple regression analysis: working memory 64
Mundt, C.: German concepts 7, 12, 138-146

naming: language disorder in dementia 166-168, 170
National Adult Reading Test: premorbid intelligence 63, 128
neologisms
  abstruse 86
  composed morphemic deviations 85
  derived morphemic deviations 84-85, 89 & Fig. 7.2
  schizophrenic 54
neural network simulation model 128, 133-135 & Figs 10.4-10.5, 145
neuroleptics: Hunt test 100
neurology of speech and language: Critchley, E. M. R. 185-194
  central disorders of language 186-187
  dynamic view of aphasias 188-190
  frontal lobes and speech 190-192
  initiation of speech 192
  inner language 190
  lateralisation of speech 187-188
  linguistic functions of the right hemisphere 187
  reception 185-186

neuropsychology of schizophrenic speech: McKenna, P. 114, 118–123
  comparisons with dysphasia 121–122 & Tab. 9.3
  conclusions 122–123
  single case studies 120–121
  studies of unselected patients 118–119
  studies using dysphasic screening batteries 119–120 & Tab. 9.2
  summary 121–122
neurotic disorders 3, 12
Newby, D.: terminology and techniques 5, 31–33
nineteenth century views on thinking and language 16–18
nodes: Mackay, D. 52–53
nonce forms 48
normal speech and language functions 139–141

obsessional symptoms 150, 153–154 & Tab. 12.1
organic disorders
  introduction 3, 8, 14
  see also brain damage
other psychiatric disorders 161–194 Part III
  language disorder in dementia: Miller, E. 163–173
  neurology of speech and language: Critchley, E. M. R. 9, 185–194
  semantics of autism: Hobson, P. 174–184
output and intention 49–50, 55
overinclusive thinking 7, 115–118 & Tab. 9.1
  diagnostic groups 116–117 & Tab. 9.1
  semantic processing and categorisation 126, 131, 134–135

parallel-distributed models: mental representations 132
paralogical in schizophrenia (Von Domarus, E.) 26
paraphasias: Lecours, A. R. & Vanier-Clement, M. 121
parole
  lésions des organes 18
  opposition to pure *langue* 48
Payne, R. W.: overinclusive thinking 116–117 & Tab. 9.1
perception: introduction 10, 13
Peritz technique: multiple pairwise comparisons 130
permeability of self 7, 9–14
personal pronouns 180–182
Peters, U. H.: sign-field disturbance 141

phatic communication (speaking without thinking): Malinowski, B. 34
phenomenological approaches: German examples 141–144
phenothiazines: Hunt test 100
philosophy of mind, insight 152–155 & Tab. 12.1
  psychopathology 155–157
phonemes (syllables) 35
  schizophrenic 54
phonetics 35–36 & Fig. 3.2
phonology 35–37 & Figs 3.2–3.3
phrenology: conceptual history 17
poetry: preverbal thinking 140
Porot, A.: term 'schizophasia' attributed to Kraepelin 82
positron emission tomography:
  comparisons of percentage blood flows 192 & Tab. 15.1
pragmatics 40–42
predicative thinking 139–140
prefrontal lobe damage: language impairment 65–66
Present State Examination (PSE) 98
Preston Psychiatric Unit for the Deaf: major syndromes 186–187
preverbal thinking 139–140
priming
  facilitation in recognition 13, 134–135
  positive and negative 167
  semantic paradigm: Spitzer, M. 144
property comparison model: categories 132
propositions: relation of words making a new meaning: Jackson, H. 20
psychoanalysis: slips of the tongue 12
psycholinguistics
  analysis of schizophrenic output 114–115
  introduction 13–14
  terminology and techniques: Newby, D. 5, 31–43
psychology of formal thought disorder: McKenna, P. 114–118, 122–123
  conclusions 122–123
  empirically oriented approaches 114–115
  summary 117–118
  theoretically oriented approaches 115–117 & Tab. 9.1
psychonomy: meaningful connections 138
psychopathology
  introduction 3–14
  philosophy of mind 155–157
  thought insertion, insight and Descarte's *cogito*: Fulford, W. 147–159
psychotherapy of hebephrenics: 'pernicious fusion' with mother: Lang, H. 142
psychotic/non-psychotic dichotomy 8, 151–152

reading: involvement of non-dominant hemisphere 187
reality assessment: German concepts of schizophrenic language disorder: Mundt, C. 138–146
reception: neurology of speech and language 185–186
'reduced redundancy' 71
references
    ambiguous 40
    'anaphoric' 39–40
religious language 141
Research Diagnostic Criteria 59, 98, 128
reversals or transpositions of letters, sounds or words 186
reverse digit span test 102, 104–105
Rochester, S. & Martin, J. R.: schizophrenic discourse 115–116
Ryle, G.: 'adhesiveness' of experience 148–149 & Fig. 12.1, 156

scales
    British Picture Vocabulary Scale (BPVS) 178–179
    Modified Rogers Scale: catatonic signs 128
    Montgomery-Asberg scale: mood state 128
    Thought Language and Communication Scale 98
    see also assessment, batteries and tests
Scheffe's procedure to compare pairs of group means 102, 105
Schilder, P.: Gestalt viewpoint 26
schizophasia: Lecours, A. 6, 81–95
    conclusions 94
    glossolalia 82, 90–94 & Fig. 7.4
    glossomania 82, 84–90 & Fig. 7.3, 94
schizophrenia
    language impairments and executive dysfunction: Morice, R. 57–69
    model of glossomanic schizophrenia 90 & Fig. 7.3
    semantic processing and categorisation: Chen, E. *et al* 126–137
    subtypes: Andreasen, N. J. C. 81–82
    term: Bleuler, E. 23–25, 81
    types I and II: Crow, T. J. 58
    see also first onset schizophrenia
schizophrenic disturbance of speech and language 45–194 Part II
    analysis: what model?: Chaika, E. 47–56
    disorder and semantic memory: Mortimer, A. *et al* 70–80
    German concepts: Mundt, C. 138–146

impairments and executive dysfunction: Morice, R. 57–69
schizophasia: Lecours, A. R. 81–95
semantic processing and categorisation: Chen, E. *et al* 126–137
syntactic processing in first-onset: Thomas, P. & Leudar, I. 96–112
thought insertion, insight and Descarte's *cogito*: Fulford, W. 147–159
thought and speech: McKenna, P. 113–125
schizophrenic terms: Andreasen, N. J. C. 81
schizophrenic thought and speech: McKenna, P. 113–125
    conclusions 122–123
    neuropsychology of schizophrenic speech 118–122
    psychology of formal thought disorder 114–118
Schneider, K.: first rank symptoms 10–11, 14
Séglas, A.: *Des Troubles de Langage chez les Aliénés* 15–16, 21–23, 27
self boundaries: introduction 7, 9–13
semantic memory: language disorder 70–79
semantic processing and categorisation: Chen, E. *et al* 7, 13, 126–137
    conclusions 135
    empirical study of categorisation in schizophrenia 128–131
    results of empirical study 129–131 & Figs 10.1–10.2
    semantic relatedness 128–129
    theoretical issues and computer simulation model 131–135
semantic store disorder: introduction 6, 78–79
semantics: meaning 36–39 & Figs 3.2–3.3
semantics of autism: Hobson, P. 9, 174–184
    conclusions 182
    meaning of 'autism' 175–177
    studies in semantics 177–182
sentences
    grammar and syntax 36–37 & Fig. 3.3
    model of sentence production: Garrett, M. 106–107
    span: working memory 63–65
Shallice, T. *et al*: errors similar to those in posterior cerebral lesions 123
shape cancelling test 102, 104–105 & Tab. 8.4
Shapiro-Wilks statistic 62
sign-field disturbance: Peters, U. H. 141

signs
  formal thought disorder 113
  introduction 3, 7
'silly sentences test' 6, 12, 75
Sims, A.: introduction 3–14
single case studies: neuropsychology 120–121
  pioneered by Chaika, E. 120
slips of the tongue 5, 12, 52–54
Spearman correlation coefficient 75, 77
speech: growth points in neurology 185–194
  frontal lobe functions 190–192
  initiation of speech 192 & Tab. 15.1
  lateralisation 187–88
  neurochemical basis 189
  propositional and non-propositional: cerebral blood flow 192 & Tab. 15.1
speech analysis: what model?: Chaika, E. 47–56
  an empirical study 50–52
  conclusions 55
  output and intention 49–50
  slips of the tongue 52–54
speech disorders
  background 1–43 Part I
  other psychiatric disorders 161–194 Part III
  schizophrenic disturbances 45–159 Part II
speech, opposite: antonymy 54, 85
Spitzer, M.: semantic priming paradigm 144
split-brain
  experiments 156
  modular nature of the mind 52
  operations 187
statistical analyses
  hypogeometric distribution 101, 110–111 App. 2
  Kolmogorov-Smirnov goodness of fit 102
  Kruskal-Wallis one-way analysis of variance 102
  Mann-Whitney test 102, 104
  Peritz technique: multiple pairwise comparisons 130
  Scheffe's procedure to compare pairs of group means 102, 105
  Shapiro-Wilks statistic 62
  Spearman correlation coefficient 77
  stem and leaf plots 60
  Z scores: Australian studies 59–60
  see also cluster, covariance, discriminant function *and* variance
Statistical Package for the Social Sciences 102

Steinbeck, J.: words 3
stem and leaf plots 60
Stengel, E.: naming errors in aphasia and dementia 166
stroke, left inferior parietal: aphasia 82
structure (form): linguistics 35–37 & Figs 3.2–3.3, 40–41
  'deep' structure: Chomsky, N. 36
studies in semantics: autism 177–182
  'emotion' words 177–178 & Fig. 14.1
  'emotion-related' words 178–180
  personal pronouns 180–182
study of written language in schizophrenia 98–105
  assessments 99–100
  complexity 102–103 & Tab. 8.2, 108–109
  controls 98–99
  demographic characteristics 99 & Tab. 8.1
  error analysis 103–104 & Tab. 8.3
  Hunt test 100–102
  measures of cognition 104–105 & Tab. 8.4
  patients 98
  results 102
summaries
  overinclusive thinking more typical of acute than chronic schizophrenia 117–118
  severe schizophrenic thought disorder related to fluent dyphasia 121
symbolic interactionism 139
symposia: psychopathology 3–4
symptoms
  first rank: Schneider, K. 10–11
  introduction 4
  obsessional 150, 153–154 & Tab. 12.1
  thought disorder as a construct 27
synapses: auto-associative network 133 & Fig. 10.4
syndromes, major: Psychiatric Unit for the Deaf at Preston 185–187
syntactic processing in first-onset schizophrenia: Thomas, P. & Leudar, I. 96–112
  discussion 105–108
  Hunt test 108–110 App. 1
  hypergeometric distribution 110–111 App. 2
  study of written language 98–105
syntax 36–38 & Figs 3.2–3.3
  schizophrenic 52–53
syntax trees
  linguistic performance: Morice, R. 6, 58–59 & Fig. 5.1, 63
  techniques: Newby, D. 5, 38 & Fig. 3.4

t-test 102
tables: differential illness-diagnosis 153–154 & Tab. 12.1 & n.
Tamlyn, D. *et al*: studies of memory impairment in schizophrenia 72–79
  discussion 78–79
  results 77–78 & Fig. 6.2
tangentionality: Andreasen, N. J. C. 85
terminology and techniques: Newby, D. 31–43
  basic definitions 31–32
  does language shape thought? 34–35 & Fig. 3.1
  levels of linguistic analysis 35–37 & Figs 3.2–3.3
  pragmatics 40–43
  relationship between thought and language 32–34
  transformational or generative grammars 37–40 Fig. 3.1
tests
  poor performance not necessarily a specific neuropsychological deficit 114
  see also Hunt, National Adult Reading, reverse digits, shape cancelling, silly sentences, *t*-test, token, Wada's carotid *and* Wisconsin card sorting *and see also* assessment, batteries *and* scales
text analysis 39–40
thalamic nuclei: speech involvement 190–191
thinking and language
  19th century 16–17
  preverbal and predicative 139–140, 143–144
Thomas, P. & Leudar, I.: syntactic processing in first-onset schizophrenia 6–7, 96–112
thought disorder: conceptual history 15–27
  early descriptions 18–20
  Masselon, R.: dementia preacox 23
  views after Masselon 23–25
thought disorder
  cognitive dysfunction 72–79
  language impairment: Bleuler, E. 57–58
  linguistic problems 70–72
  speech disorder: Chaika, E. 96
thought insertion, insight and Descartes' *cogito* 7–8, 11, 147–159
  conclusions 157–158
  Descartes' *cogito* and thought insertion 148–150 & Fig. 12.1
  philosophy of mind and insight 152–155 & Tab. 1

psychopathology and the philosophy of mind 155–157
thought insertion and insight 150–152
Thought Language and Communication Scale 98
thought and language relationships
  conceptual history 17–18
  does language shape thought? 34–35 Fig. 3.1
  Jackson's views 20–21
  terminology and techniques 32–34
token test (de Renzi, E. & Vognolo, L. A.): comprehension of syntax 62–64 & Tab. 5.2, 169
Tower of London: forward planning: Shallice, T. 63
'trade-offs': linguistic variables 59–61
transcortical sensory aphasia 165–166
transformational or generative grammars 37–39 & Fig. 3.4
two-stage feature comparison model: semantic processing 132
typing errors 185

unconscious processes: slips of the tongue 52–54
use/structure interface 36 Fig. 3.2, 40–41
utterances, glossomanic 86–90

variables, linguistic 59–62 & Tabs 5.1–5.2
verbigerations: Séglas, J. 22
volitional lapses 52, 55
  introduction 5
Von Domarus, E.: schizophrenic thinking 26
vowels: perception better than consonants 187

Wada's carotid amytal test 188
Webster's Third New International Dictionary: definition of language 32
Wernicke's aphasia
  glossolalia 90–91, 94
  hormonal or neurotransmitter hypofunction 188
  introduction 6
  language impairment in dementia 165–166
  language impairment and executive dysfunction 57, 62
  neologisms 86, 89
  prognosis 189
  specific nature 189–190
Whorf's language relativism 140
Wing, L.: autism 175

Wisconsin card sorting test: cognitive flexibility 63, 66
word meanings 174–175
words
  linguistic elements 35
  'emotion' (autism) 177–178 & Fig. 14.1
  'emotion-related' (autism) 178–180
  Steinbeck, J. 3
  see also *langue* and *parole*
  Hugo, V. 15
working memory
  executive impairment 63–67 & Tabs 5.4–5.6
  introduction 7, 12
  syntactic processing 101–102, 104–106 & Tab. 8.4
  introduction 6–7
  study in schizophrenia 98–108
  two-way interaction between thought and language 34–35 & Fig. 3.1

Z scores: Australian studies 59–60
Zangwill, O. L. *Speech and the minor hemisphere* 188